BEYOND PRICE

Beyond Price

Essays on Birth and Death

J. David Velleman

OpenBook Publishers

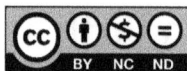

ISBN Paperback: 978-1-78374-167-0
ISBN Hardback: 978-1-78374-168-7
ISBN Digital (PDF): 978-1-78374-169-4
ISBN Digital ebook (epub): 978-1-78374-170-0
ISBN Digital ebook (mobi): 978-1-78374-171-7
DOI: 10.11647/OBP.0061

Cover image: Gustav Klimt, *Die drei Lebensalter der Frau* (1905). Wikimedia, http://commons.wikimedia.org/wiki/File:Gustav_Klimt_020.jpg

All paper used by Open Book Publishers is SFI (Sustainable Forestry Initiative) and PEFC (Programme for the Endorsement of Forest Certification Schemes) certified.

Printed in the United Kingdom and United States by Lightning Source for Open Book Publishers (Cambridge, UK).

Contents

1. Introduction

Beyond Price collects my essays in bioethics, most of which are unified by a rejection of the prevailing egoistic voluntarism about ending one's own life and creating new ones — that is, about suicide and procreation.

Many now believe that it is not only permissible but virtuous to "take control" of one's death and to exercise that control when life is no longer "worth it". Feature articles in the press celebrate the courage of people who commit suicide because the benefits of longevity no longer repay them for the burdens of old age. And society is happy to be relieved of responsibility for euthanasia by those who take the initiative to self-euthanize.

In three essays ("Against the Right to Die?", "A Right of Self-Termination?", and "Beyond Price"), I argue that having control over one's death is itself a burden, and that the calculation of benefits and burdens is in any case inadequate to guide a decision in which the value of the person is at stake. I ultimately arrive at the conclusion that the choice of death should be guided not by self-interest but by love — which, I believe, regards the intact rational capacity to make the choice as a reason for not making it, at least not yet.

Procreation is another site for the self-interested assertion of will, as infertile couples and single women create children by buying gametes from anonymous strangers. Although a large segment of our society denies that whether to abort a pregnancy is a private decision, there is oddly no party platform denying that it's a private decision whether to have a child. I say "oddly" because what makes the privacy of abortion so controversial — that is, disagreement as to whether there is another person involved — should make it uncontroversial that procreation is not private. There obviously is another person involved: the child.

No doubt, the living child is left out of account because it receives what the aborted fetus is denied, the so-called gift of life. I contend that life is not

http://dx.doi.org/10.11647/OBP.0061.01

a gift, and that "giving" it to a child is wrong if the child will be severed from half of its ancestry. Defending this contention requires some careful reasoning about personal identity and nonexistence, which I undertake over the course of four essays ("Family History" and the three parts of "Persons in Prospect").

These seven essays are informed by Kantian and Aristotelian thought, though they are hardly faithful to the theories of Kant or Aristotle. The operative Kantian thought is expressed in this volume's title. The thought is that rational nature is "beyond price" in the sense that it must not be weighed against self-interest. I expand on this thought by arguing that rational nature merits not only Kantian respect but also love, which is continuous with respect, in my view. The Aristotelian thought is that a person's good is that which it makes sense to want out of friendship-love for the person, and what it makes sense to want out of love is that the person fully express his or her capacities.

The subsequent three essays in the collection are about the harm of death. Over the twenty-odd years between the earliest paper in the collection ("Well-Being and Time") and the latest ("Dying"), my attitude toward death has gradually changed. I no longer think that the question of how to feel about death has a single right answer. Although I don't point it out in the essays themselves, Part III of "Persons in Prospect" provides the foundations for my conclusion in "Dying" that a single answer is unnecessary.

Although bioethics is usually classified under the heading of applied ethics, these essays are not "applied" in the usual sense. I don't propose or defend any particular policies, much less legislation, on the issues that I discuss. Nor do I deal with the specifics of decision-making in particular cases. Although I argue that, other things being equal, children should know and be reared by their biological parents, I don't go into the many possible degrees of knowledge, or the possible variations of child-rearing arrangements. In the case of assisted suicide, I even argue that philosophy cannot penetrate to the level of guiding particular decisions.

In writing about these topics, I aim rather to figure out how to think about them, not what to think at the level of practical application. My topic is not metaethics, it's not applied ethics, and it's not normative ethics, either — not, at least, if normative ethics is the comparative study of normative theories such as utilitarianism, Kant's categorical imperative, and virtue ethics. I think of my topic as the foundations of applied ethics, the goal being to better understand the underlying notions of personhood, parenthood, autonomy, well-being, and so on, with an eye to how those notions will apply to practice in general.

Insofar as my views have practical consequences, they have sometimes been described as conservative, in the political sense of the word. For what it's worth, my political sympathies are liberal. No doubt they influence my philosophical views, but philosophy sometimes leads me to conclusions that, however liberal in my eyes, are disdained by members of my political party. Those are the conclusions to which I prefer to devote my intellectual efforts, because they are more interesting to me than the ones on which I follow the party line. To that extent, I am a contrarian — not because I seek out perverse conclusions but rather because I find philosophy most interesting when it leads to conclusions that seem perverse, and I choose to write about what interests me. As Bertrand Russell said, "The point of philosophy is to start with something so simple as not to seem worth stating, and to end with something so paradoxical that no one will believe it."[1] Arguing for the obvious is not worthy of a philosopher's time.

The last essay in the collection is about life-writing — biography and autobiography — and it concludes with some autobiography of my own. I have the nagging sense that my mixing autobiography with philosophy, always self-indulgent, is sometimes unfair. I commit the fallacy of *argumentum ad misericordiam* by revealing unfortunate parts of my life history, as if soliciting philosophical agreement by appealing for personal sympathy. All I can say in my own defense is that I have included a lot of happy autobiography in my work, as in "Family History", and that I actually regard all of my writing as autobiographical. Although I write about what it is like to be a human being, I am always aware of writing only about what it is like for me.

I have many debts to students and colleagues who commented on these papers and to institutions that invited me to present them. Those debts are acknowledged in the first footnote of each chapter (which also indicates whether I have made revisions beyond minor editorial emendations). I am indebted to my copyeditor, Katherine Duke, for transforming an unruly mob of documents into a well-behaved manuscript. And it has been a pleasure to work with Rupert Gatti, Alessandra Tosi, and Ben Fried on my second book with Open Book Publishers.

---

1   *The Philosophy of Logical Atomism* (Abingdon: Routledge Classics, 2010), p. 20.

2. Against the Right to Die[1]

In this chapter I argue that a widely recognized right to die would have the paradoxical effect of harming some people who never exercise it as well as some who exercise it and are better off for doing so. Even more paradoxically, recognition of such a right would make it difficult if not impossible to define a class of people to whom it should be accorded in practice.

My arguments do not lead me to conclude that there is no universal right to die. Maybe there are some rights whose recognition is harmful to many people and whose proper subjects cannot practically be identified. Moreover, I do believe that some people are morally entitled to help in dying. What I do not believe is that this entitlement can or should be recognized as a universal right.

I

Although I believe in our obligation to facilitate some deaths, I want to dissociate myself from some of the arguments that are frequently offered for such an obligation. These arguments, like many arguments in medical

---

1 The present chapter has been supplemented and in many respects superseded by my "A Right of Self-Termination?", chapter 3 of this volume, and "Beyond Price", chapter 4. It is an extensively revised version of a paper that was originally published in *The Journal of Medicine & Philosophy* 17 (1992): 665-681, http://dx.doi.org/10.1093/jmp/17.6.665. A subsequent version appeared in the second edition of *Ethics in Practice: An Anthology*, ed. High LaFollette (Chichester: John Wiley & Sons, 2014), pp. 96-100. That chapter began as a comment on a paper by Dan W. Brock, presented at the Central Division of the APA in 1991. See his "Voluntary Active Euthanasia" (*The Hastings Center Report* 22 [1992]: 10-22; reprinted in *Life and Death: Philosophical Essays in Biomedical Ethics* [Cambridge: Cambridge University Press, 1993], pp. 202-234). I received help in writing that paper from Dan Brock, Elizabeth Anderson, David Hills, Yale Kamisar, and Patricia White.

http://dx.doi.org/10.11647/OBP.0061.02

ethics, rely on terms borrowed from Kantian moral theory — terms such as 'dignity' and 'autonomy'. Various kinds of life-preserving treatment are said to violate a patient's dignity or to detain him in an undignified state; and the patient's right of autonomy is said to require that we respect his competent and considered wishes, including a wish to die. There may or may not be some truth in each of these claims. Yet when we evaluate such claims, we must not assume that terms like 'dignity' and 'autonomy' always express the same concepts, or carry the same normative force, as they do in a particular moral theory.

When Kant speaks, for example, of the dignity that belongs to persons by virtue of their rational nature, and that places them beyond all price,[2] he is not invoking anything that requires the ability to walk unaided, to feed oneself, or to control one's bowels. Hence the dignity invoked in discussions of medical ethics — a status supposedly threatened by physical deterioration and dependency — cannot be the status whose claim on our moral concern is so fundamental to Kantian thought. We must therefore ask whether this other sort of dignity, whatever it may be, embodies a value that's equally worthy of protection.

My worry, in particular, is that the word 'dignity' is sometimes used to dignify, so to speak, our culture's obsession with independence, physical strength, and youth. To my mind, the dignity defined by these values — a dignity that is ultimately incompatible with *being cared for* at all — is a dignity not worth having.[3]

I have similar worries about the values expressed by the phrase 'patient autonomy', for there are two very different senses in which a person's autonomy can become a value for us. On the one hand, we can obey the categorical imperative, by declining to act for reasons that we could not rationally propose as valid for all rational beings, including those who are affected by our action, such as the patient. What we value in that case is the patent's *capacity* for self-determination, and we value it in a particular way — namely, by according it *respect*. We respect the patient's autonomy by regarding the necessity of sharing our reasons with him, among others, as a constraint on what decisions we permit ourselves to reach.

---

2   Immanuel Kant, *Groundwork of the Metaphysic of Morals*, trans. H. J. Paton (New York: Harper & Row, 1964), p. 102.

3   Here I echo some excellent remarks on the subject by Felicia Ackerman in "No, Thanks, I Don't Want to Die with Dignity", *Providence Journal-Bulletin*, April 19, 1990. I discuss the issue of "dying with dignity" in "A Right of Self-Termination?".

On the other hand, we can value the patient's autonomy by making it our goal to maximize his effective options. What we value, in that case, is not the patient's capacity but his *opportunities* for self-determination — his having choices to make and the means with which to implement them; and we value these opportunities for self-determination by regarding them as *goods* — as objects of desire and pursuit rather than respect.

These two ways of valuing autonomy are fundamentally different. Respecting people's autonomy, in the Kantian sense, is not just a matter of giving them effective options. To make our own decisions only for reasons that we could rationally share with others is not necessarily to give *them* decisions to make, nor is it to give them the means to implement their actual decisions.[4]

As with the term 'dignity', then, we must not assume that the term 'autonomy' is always being used in the sense made familiar by Kantian moral theory; and we must therefore ask ourselves what sort of autonomy is being invoked, and whether it is indeed something worthy of our moral concern. I believe that, as with the term 'dignity', the answer to the latter question may be "no" in some cases, including the case of the right to die.

II

Despite my qualms about the use of Kantian language to justify euthanasia, I do believe that euthanasia can be justified, and on Kantian grounds. In particular, I believe that respect for a person's dignity, properly conceived, can require us to facilitate his death when that dignity is being irremediably compromised. I also believe, however, that a person's dignity can be so compromised only by circumstances that are likely to compromise his capacity for fully rational and autonomous decision-making. So although I do not favor euthanizing people against their wills, of course, neither do I favor a policy of euthanizing people for the sake of deferring to their wills, since I think that people's wills are usually impaired in the circumstances required to make euthanasia permissible. The sense in which I oppose a right to die, then, is that I oppose treating euthanasia as a protected option for the patient.

---

4   I discuss this issue further in "Love as a Moral Emotion", *Ethics* 109 (1999): 338-374, pp. 356-358, esp. nn. 69, 72. That paper was reprinted in *Self to Self: Selected Essays* (New York: Cambridge University Press, 2005), pp. 70-109.

One reason for my opposition is the associated belief (also Kantian) that so long as patients are fully competent to exercise an option of being euthanized, their doing so would be immoral, in the majority of cases, because their dignity as persons would still be intact. I discuss this argument elsewhere, but I do not return to it in the present paper.[5] In this paper I discuss a second reason for opposing euthanasia as a protected option for the patient. This reason, unlike the first, is consequentialist.

What consequentialist arguments could there be against giving the option of euthanasia to patients? One argument, of course, would be that giving this option to patients, even under carefully defined conditions, would entail providing euthanasia to some patients for whom it would be a harm rather than a benefit.[6] This argument depends on the assumption that patients granted a right to die might mistakenly choose to die when they would be better off living. My argument makes no such assumption.

In order to demonstrate that I am not primarily worried about mistaken requests to die, I shall assume, from this point forward, that patients are infallible, and that euthanasia would therefore be chosen only by those for whom it would be a benefit. Even so, I believe, the recognition of a right to die would harm many patients, by increasing their autonomy in a sense that is not only un-Kantian but also highly undesirable.

This belief is sometimes expressed in public debate, although it is rarely developed in any detail. Here, for example, is Yale Kamisar's argument against "Euthanasia Legislation":[7]

> Is this the kind of choice ... that we want to offer a gravely ill person? Will we not sweep up, in the process, some who are not really tired of life, but think others are tired of them; some who do not really want to die, but who feel they should not live on, because to do so when there looms the legal alternative of euthanasia is to do a selfish or a cowardly act? Will not some feel an obligation to have themselves "eliminated"...?

Note that these considerations do not, strictly speaking, militate against euthanasia itself. Rather, they militate against a particular decision procedure for euthanasia — namely, the procedure of placing the choice of euthanasia in the patient's hands. What Kamisar is questioning in this

---

5 See "A Right of Self-Termination?" and "Beyond Price", chapters 3 and 4 of this volume.

6 See Yale Kamisar, "Euthanasia Legislation: Some Non-Religious Objections", in *Euthanasia and the Right to Death: The Case for Voluntary Euthanasia*, ed. A. B. Downing (New York: Humanities Press, 1970), pp. 85-133.

7 Ibid., p. 95.

passage is, not the practice of helping some patients to die, but rather the practice of asking them to choose whether to die. The feature of legalized euthanasia that troubles him is precisely its being an option offered to patients — the very feature for which it's touted, by its proponents, as an enhancement of patients' autonomy. Kamisar's remark thus betrays the suspicion that this particular enhancement of one's autonomy is not to be welcomed.

But what exactly is the point of Kamisar's rhetorical questions? The whole purpose of giving people choices, surely, is to allow those choices to be determined by their reasons and preferences rather than ours. Kamisar may think that finding one's life tiresome is a good reason for dying, whereas thinking that others find one tiresome is not. But if others honestly think otherwise, why should we stand in their way? Whose life is it anyway?

III

A theoretical framework for addressing this question can be found in Thomas Schelling's book *The Strategy of Conflict*,[8] and in Gerald Dworkin's paper "Is More Choice Better than Less?"[9] These authors have shown that our intuitions about the value of options are often mistaken, and their work can help us to understand the point of arguments like Kamisar's.

We are inclined to think that, unless we are likely to make mistakes about whether to exercise an option (as I am assuming we are not), the value of having the option is as high as the value of exercising it and no lower than zero. Exercising an option can of course be worse than nothing, if it causes harm. But if we are not prone to mistakes, then we will not exercise a harmful option; and we tend to think that simply *having* the unexercised option cannot be harmful. And insofar as exercising an option would make us better off than we are, having the option must have made us better off than we were before we had it — or so we tend to think.

What Schelling showed, however, is that having an option can be harmful even if we do not exercise it and — more surprisingly — even if we exercise it and gain by doing so. Schelling's examples of this phenomenon were drawn primarily from the world of negotiation, where the only way to induce one's

---

8   Cambridge, MA: Harvard University Press, 1960.
9   *Midwest Studies in Philosophy* 7 (1982): 47-61.

opponent to settle for less may be by proving that one doesn't have the option of giving him more. Schelling pointed out that in such circumstances, a lack of options can be an advantage. The union leader who cannot persuade his membership to approve a pay cut, or the ambassador who cannot contact his head of state for a change of brief, negotiates from a position of strength, whereas the negotiator for whom all concessions are possible deals from weakness. If the rank and file give their leader the option of offering a pay cut, then management may not settle for anything less, whereas they might have settled for less if he hadn't had the option of making the offer. The union leader will then have to decide whether to take the option and reach an agreement or to leave the option and call a strike. But no matter which of these outcomes would make him better off, choosing it will still leave him worse off than he would have been if he had never had the option at all.

Dworkin has expanded on Schelling's point by exploring other respects in which options can be undesirable. Just as options can subject one to pressure from an opponent in negotiation, for example, they can subject one to pressure from other sources as well. The night cashier in a convenience store doesn't want the option of opening the safe — and not because he fears that he'd make mistakes about when to open it. It is precisely because the cashier would know when he'd better open the safe that his having the option would make him an attractive target for robbers; and it's because having the option would make him a target for robbers that he'd be better off without it. The cashier who finds himself opening the safe at gunpoint can consistently think that he's doing what's best while wishing that he'd never been given the option of doing it.

Options can be undesirable, then, because they subject one to various kinds of pressure; but they can be undesirable for other reasons, too. Offering someone an alternative to the status quo makes two outcomes possible for him, but neither of them is the outcome that was possible before. He can now choose the status quo or choose the alternative, but he can no longer *have* the status quo without *choosing* it. And having the status quo by default may have been what was best for him, even though choosing the status quo is now worst. If I invite you to a dinner party, I leave you the possibilities of choosing to come or choosing to stay away; but I deprive you of something that you otherwise would have had — namely, the possibility of being absent from my table by default, as you are on all other occasions. Surely, preferring to accept an invitation is consistent with wishing you had never received it. These attitudes are consistent because refusing to attend a party is a different outcome from *not* attending without having to refuse; and even if the former of these outcomes is worse than attending, the latter may still have been better. Having choices can thus deprive one of desirable outcomes whose desirability depends on their being unchosen.

The offer of an option can also be undesirable because of what it expresses. To offer a student the option of receiving remedial instruction after class is to imply that he is not keeping up. If the student needs help but doesn't know it, the offer may clue him in. But even if the student does not need any help to begin with, the offer may so undermine his confidence that he will need help before long. In the latter case, the student may ultimately benefit from accepting the offer, even though he would have been better off not receiving it at all.

Note that in each of these cases, a person can be harmed by having a choice even if he chooses what's best for him. Once the option of offering a concession has undermined one's bargaining position, once the option of opening the safe has made one the target of a robbery, once the invitation to a party has eliminated the possibility of absence by default, once the offer of remedial instruction has implied that one needs it — in short, once one has been offered a problematic choice — one's situation has already been altered for the worse, and choosing what's best cannot remedy the harm that one has already suffered. Choosing what's best in these cases is simply a way of cutting one's losses.

Note, finally, that we cannot always avoid burdening people with options by offering them a second-order option as to which options they are to be offered. If issuing you an invitation to dinner would put you in an awkward position, then asking you whether you want to be invited would usually do so as well; if offering you the option of remedial instruction would send you a message, then so would asking you whether you'd like that option. In order to avoid doing harm, then, we are sometimes required, not only to withhold options, but also to take the initiative for withholding them.

IV

Of course, the options that I have discussed can also be unproblematic for many people in many circumstances. Sometimes one has good reason to welcome a dinner invitation or an offer of remedial instruction. Similarly, some patients will welcome the option of euthanasia, and rightly so. The problem is how to offer the option only to those patients who will have reason to welcome it. Arguments like Kamisar's are best understood, I think, as warning that the option of euthanasia may unavoidably be offered to some who will be harmed simply by having the option, even if they go on to choose what is best.

I think that the option of euthanasia may harm some patients in all of the ways canvassed above; but I will focus my attention on only a few of those ways. The most important way in which the option of euthanasia may harm patients, I think, is that it will deny them the possibility of staying alive by default.

Now, the idea of surviving by default will be anathema to existentialists, who will insist that the choice between life and death is a choice that we have to make every day, perhaps every moment.[10] Yet even if there is a deep, philosophical sense in which we do continually choose to go on living, it is not reflected in our ordinary self-understanding. That is, we do not ordinarily think of ourselves or others as continually rejecting the option of suicide and staying alive by choice. Thus, even if the option of euthanasia won't alter a patient's existential situation, it will certainly alter the way in which his situation is generally perceived. And changes in the perception of a patient's situation will be sufficient to produce many of the problems that Schelling and Dworkin have described, since those problems are often created not just by *having* options but by *being seen* to have them.

Once a person is given the choice between life and death, he will rightly be perceived as the agent of his own survival. Whereas his existence is ordinarily viewed as a given for him — as a fixed condition with which he must cope — formally offering him the option of euthanasia will cause his existence thereafter to be viewed as his doing.

The problem with this perception is that if others regard you as choosing a state of affairs, they will hold you responsible for it; and if they hold you responsible for a state of affairs, they can ask you to justify it. Hence, if people ever come to regard you as existing by choice, they may expect you to justify your continued existence. If your daily arrival in the office is interpreted as meaning that you have once again declined to kill yourself, you may feel obliged to arrive with an answer to the question "Why not?"

I think that our perception of one another's existence as a given is so deeply ingrained that we can hardly imagine what life would be like without it. When someone shows impatience or displeasure with us, we jokingly say, "Well, excuse me for living!" But imagine that it were no joke;

---

10 The locus classicus for this point is, of course, Albert Camus's essay "The Myth of Sisyphus", in *The Myth of Sisyphus and Other Essays*, trans. Justin O'Brien (New York: Vintage Books, 1956), pp. 88-91.

imagine that living were something for which one might reasonably be thought to need an excuse. The burden of justifying one's existence might make existence unbearable — and hence unjustifiable.

V

I assume that people care, and are right to care, about whether they can justify their choices to others. Of course, this concern can easily seem like slavishness or neurotic insecurity; but it should not be dismissed too lightly. Our ability to justify our choices to the people around us is what enables us to sustain the role of rational agent in our dealings with them; and it is therefore essential to our remaining, in their eyes, eligible partners in cooperation and conversation, or appropriate objects of respect.

Retaining one's status as a person among others is especially important to those who are ill or infirm. I imagine that when illness or infirmity denies one the rewards of independent activity, then the rewards of personal intercourse may be all that make life worth living. To the ill or infirm, then, the ability to sustain the role of rational person may rightly seem essential to retaining what remains of value in life. Being unable to account for one's choices may seem to entail the risk of being perceived as unreasonable — as not worth reasoning with — and consequently being cut off from meaningful intercourse with others, which is life's only remaining consolation.

Forcing a patient to take responsibility for his continued existence may therefore be tantamount to confronting him with the following prospect: unless he can explain, to the satisfaction of others, why he chooses to exist, his only remaining reasons for existence may vanish.

VI

Unfortunately, our culture is extremely hostile to any attempt at justifying an existence of passivity and dependence. The burden of proof will lie heavily on the patient who thinks that his terminal illness or chronic disability is not a sufficient reason for dying.

What is worse, the people with whom a patient wants to maintain intercourse, and to whom he therefore wants to justify his choices, are often in a position to incur several financial and emotional costs from any prolongation of his life. Many of the reasons in favor of his death are therefore likely to be exquisitely salient in their minds. I believe that some of these people may actively pressure the patient to exercise the option of dying. (Students who hear me say this usually object that no one would ever do such a thing. My reply is that no one would ever do such a thing as abuse his own children or parents — except that some people do).

In practice, however, friends and relatives of a patient will not have to utter a word of encouragement, much less exert any overt pressure, once the option of euthanasia is offered. For in the discussion of a subject so hedged by taboos and inhibitions, the patient will have to make some assumptions about what they think and how they feel, irrespective of what they say.[11] And the rational assumption for him to make will be that they are especially sensible of the considerations in favor of his exercising the option.

Thus, even if a patient antecedently believes that his life is worth living, he may have good reason to assume that many of the people around him do not, and that his efforts to convince them will be frustrated by prevailing opinions about lives like his, or by the biases inherent in their perspective. Indeed, he can reasonably assume that the offer of euthanasia is itself an expression of attitudes that are likely to frustrate his efforts to justify declining it. He can therefore assume that his refusal to take the option of euthanasia will threaten his standing as a rational person in the eyes of friends and family, thereby threatening the very things that make his life worthwhile. This patient may rationally judge that he's better off taking the option of euthanasia, even though he would have been best off not having the option at all.

Establishing a right to die in our culture may thus be like establishing a right to duel in a culture obsessed with personal honor.[12] If someone defended the right to duel by arguing that a duel is a private transaction between consenting adults, he would have missed the point of laws against dueling. What makes it rational for someone to throw down or pick up a gauntlet may be the social costs of choosing not to, costs that result from failing to duel only if one fails to duel by choice. Such costs disappear if the choice of dueling can be taken off the table. By eliminating the option of dueling (if we can), we eliminate the reasons that make it rational for

---

11 See Thomas C. Schelling, "Strategic Relationships in Dying", in *Choice and Consequence: Perspectives of an Errant Economist* (Cambridge, MA: Harvard University Press, 1984), pp. 147-157.

12 For this analogy, see Lance K. Stell, "Dueling and the Right to Life", *Ethics* 90 (1979): 7-26. Stell argues — implausibly, in my view — that one has the right to die for the same reason that one has a right to duel.

people to duel in most cases. To restore the option of dueling would be to give people reasons for dueling that they didn't previously have. Similarly, I believe, to offer the option of dying may be to give people new reasons for dying.

VII

Do not attempt to refute this argument against the right to die by labeling it paternalistic. The argument is not paternalistic — at least, not in any derogatory sense of the word. Paternalism, in the derogatory sense, is the policy of saving people from self-inflicted harms by denying them options that they might exercise unwisely. Such a policy is distasteful because it expresses a lack of respect for others' ability to make their own decisions.

But my argument is not paternalistic in this sense. My reason for withholding the option of euthanasia is not that others cannot be trusted to exercise it wisely. On the contrary, I have assumed from the outset that patients will be infallible in their deliberations. What I have argued is not that people to whom we offer the option of euthanasia might harm themselves but rather that in offering them this option, *we* will do them harm. My argument is therefore based on a simple policy of nonmalfeasance rather than on the policy of paternalism. I am arguing that we must not harm others by giving them choices, not that we must withhold the choices from them lest they harm themselves.

Of course, harming some people by giving them choices may be unavoidable if we cannot withhold those choices from them without unjustly withholding the same choices from others. If a significant number of patients were both competent and morally entitled to choose euthanasia, then we might be obligated to make that option available even if, in doing so, we would inevitably give it to some who would be harmed by having it. Consider here a closely related option.[13] People are morally entitled to refuse treatment, because they are morally entitled not to be drugged, punctured, or irradiated against their wills — in short, not to be assaulted. Protecting the right not to be assaulted entails giving some patients what amounts to the option of ending their lives. And for some subset of these patients, having the option of ending their lives by refusing treatment

---

13 The analogy is suggested, in the form of an objection to my arguments, by Dan Brock in "Voluntary Active Euthanasia".

may be just as harmful as having the option of electing active euthanasia. Nevertheless, these harms must be tolerated as an inevitable byproduct of protecting the right not to be assaulted.

Similarly, if I believed that people had a moral right to end their lives, I would not entertain consequentialist arguments against protecting that right. But I don't believe in such a moral right, for reasons to which I have briefly alluded but cannot fully expound in this chapter. My willingness to entertain the arguments expounded here thus depends on reasons that are explained elsewhere.[14]

VIII

I have been assuming, in deference to existentialists, that a right to die would not alter the options available to a patient but would, at most, alter the social perception of his options. What would follow, however, if we assumed that death was not ordinarily a genuine option? In that case, offering someone the choice of euthanasia would not only cause his existence to be perceived as his responsibility; it would actually cause his existence to become his responsibility for the first time. And this new responsibility might entail new and potentially burdensome obligations.

That options can be undesirable because they entail obligations is a familiar principle in one area of everyday life — namely, the practice of offering, accepting, and declining gifts and favors. When we decline a gift or a favor that someone has spontaneously offered, we deny him an option: the option of providing us with a particular benefit. And our reason for declining is often that he could not have the option of providing the benefit without being obligated to exercise that option. Indeed, we sometimes feel obligated, on our part, to decline a benefit precisely in order to prevent someone from being obligated, on his part, to provide it.[15] We thus recognize that giving or leaving someone the option of providing a benefit to us may be a way of harming him, by burdening him with an obligation.

---

14 See my "Right of Self-Termination?" and "Beyond Price", chapters 3 and 4 of this volume.

15 Of course, there are many other reasons for declining gifts and favors, such as pride, embarrassment, or a desire not to be in someone else's debt. My point is simply that there are cases in which these reasons are absent and a very different reason is present — namely, our desire not to burden someone else with obligations.

When we decline a gift or favor, our would-be benefactor sometimes protests in language similar to that used by proponents of the right to die. "I know what I'm doing", he says, "and no one is twisting my arm. It's my money [or whatever], and I want you to have it." If he's unaware of the lurking allusion, he might even put it like this: "Whose money is it, anyway?"

Well, it is his money (or whatever); and we do believe that he's entitled to dispose of his money as he likes. Yet his right of personal autonomy in disposing of his money doesn't always require that we let him dispose of it on us. We are entitled — and, as I have suggested, sometimes obligated — to restrict his freedom in spending his money for our benefit, insofar as that freedom may entail burdensome obligations.

The language in which favors are declined is equally interesting as that in which they are offered. What we often say when declining a favor is, "I can't let you do that for me: it would be too much to ask." The phrase 'too much to ask' is interesting because it is used only when we haven't in fact asked for anything. Precisely because the favor in question would be too much to ask, we haven't asked for it, and now our prospective benefactor is offering it spontaneously. Why, then, do we give our reason for not having solicited the favor as a reason for declining when it's offered unsolicited?

The answer, I think, is that we recognize how little distance there is between permitting someone to do us a favor and asking him to do it. Because leaving someone the option of doing us a favor can place him under an obligation to do it, it has all the consequences of asking for the favor. To say "I'm leaving you the option of helping me, but I'm not asking you to help" is to draw a distinction without a difference, since options can be just as burdensome as requests.

IX

Clearly, a patient's decision to die will sometimes be a gift or a favor bestowed on loved ones whose financial or emotional resources are being drained by his condition. And clearly, death is the sort of gift that one might well want to decline, by denying others the option of giving it. Yet protections for the option of euthanasia would in effect protect the option of giving this gift, and they would thereby prevent the prospective beneficiaries from declining it. Recognizing a right to die would thus be tantamount to adopting the view that death is never too much to ask.

I don't pretend to understand fully the ethics of gifts and favors. It's one of those subjects that gets neglected in philosophical ethics, perhaps because it has more to do with the supererogatory than the obligatory. One question that puzzles me is whether we are permitted to restrict people's freedom to benefit us in ways that require no active participation on our part. Someone cannot successfully give us a gift, in most cases, unless we cooperate by taking it into our possession; and denying someone the option of giving us a gift usually consists of refusing to do our part in the transaction. But what about cases in which someone can do us a good turn without any cooperation from us? To what extent are we entitled to decline the favor by means of restrictions on his behavior rather than omissions in ours?

Another question, of course, is whether we wouldn't, in fact, play some part in the deaths of patients who received socially sanctioned euthanasia. Would a medically assisted or supervised death be a gift that we truly took no part in accepting? What if "we" — the intended beneficiary of the gift — were society as a whole, the body that recognized the right to die and perhaps even trained physicians in its implementation? Surely, establishing the right to die is tantamount to saying, to those who might contemplate dying for the social good, that such favors will never be refused.

These considerations, inconclusive though they are, show how the theoretical framework developed by Schelling and Dworkin might support remarks like Kamisar's about patients' "obligation to have themselves 'eliminated'". The worry that a right to die would become an obligation to die is of a piece with other worries about euthanasia, not in itself, but as a problematic option for the patient.

X

As I have said, I favor euthanasia in some cases. And of course, I believe that euthanasia must not be administered to competent patients without their consent. To that extent, I think that the option of dying will have to be presented to some patients, so that they can receive the benefit of a good death.

On the basis of the foregoing arguments, however, I doubt whether we can formulate a general definition that distinguishes the circumstances in which the option of dying would be beneficial from those in which it would be harmful. The factors that make an option problematic are too subtle and too various to be defined in general rules. How will the option of euthanasia be perceived by the patient and his loved ones? How will it affect the relations among them? Is he likely to fear being spurned for declining the option? Would he exercise the option merely as a favor to them? And are they genuinely willing to accept that favor? Sensitivity to these and related questions could never be incorporated into a rule defining conditions under which the option must be offered.

Insofar as I am swayed by the foregoing arguments, then, I am inclined to think that society should at most permit, and never require, health professionals to offer the option of euthanasia or to grant patients' requests for it. We can probably define some conditions under which the option should never be offered; but we are not in a position to define conditions under which it should always be offered; and so we can at most define a legal permission rather than a legal requirement to offer it. The resulting rule would leave caregivers free to withhold the option whenever they see fit, even if it is explicitly and spontaneously requested. And so long as caregivers are permitted to withhold the option of euthanasia, patients will not be accorded a right to die.

XI

The foregoing arguments make me worry even about an explicitly formulated permission for the practice of euthanasia, since an explicit law or regulation to this effect would already invite patients, and hence potentially pressure them, to request that the permission be exercised in their case. I feel most comfortable with a policy of permitting euthanasia by default — that is, by a tacit failure to enforce the institutional rules that currently serve as barriers to justified euthanasia, or a gradual elimination of those rules without fanfare. The best public policy of euthanasia, I sometimes think, is no policy at all.

This suggestion will surely strike some readers as scandalous, because of the trust that it would place in the individual judgment of physicians and patients. But I suspect that to place one's life in the hands of another person, as one does today when placing oneself in the care of a physician, may simply be to enter a relationship in which such trust is essential, because it cannot be replaced or even underwritten by institutional guarantees. Although I do not share the conventional view that advances in medical technology have outrun our moral understanding of how they should be applied, I am indeed tempted to think they have outrun the capacity of rules to regulate their application. I am therefore tempted to think that public policy regulating the relation between physician and patient should be weak and vague by design; and that insofar as the aim of medical ethics is to strengthen or sharpen such policy, medical ethics itself is a bad idea.

3. A Right of Self-Termination?[1]

Getting cancer changed my feelings about people who smoke.

I remember hearing a fellow philosopher expound, with a wave of his cigarette, on his right to choose whether to live and die smoking, or to quit and merely survive. I was just beginning a year of chemotherapy, and mere survival sounded pretty good to me. But I was the visiting speaker, and my hosts were unaware of my diagnosis. Several of them lit up after dinner as we listened to their colleague's disquisition — they with amused familiarity, I with an outrage that surprised even me and would have baffled them, if I had dared to express it. That I didn't dare is a cause for regret even now, ten years after the fact.

1   Originally published in *Ethics* 109 (1999): 606-628, http://dx.doi.org/10.1086/233924; reprinted in *Death, Dying and the Ending of Life,* ed. Margaret P. Battin, Leslie P. Francis, and Bruce M. Landesman (Aldershot: Ashgate, 2007), pp. 275-292. Work on this chapter was supported by a fellowship from the National Endowment for the Humanities and by a sabbatical leave from the College of Literature, Science, and the Arts at the University of Michigan. An earlier and very different version was presented to the philosophy department and the Center for Ethics and Humanities in the Life Sciences at Michigan State University. I received helpful comments on that version from Elizabeth Anderson and Stephen Darwall, both of whom have also contributed significantly to my thinking on this subject through their published work. I also received comments from Bette Crigger and an anonymous referee for *The Hastings Center Report.* For comments on the present version, I am grateful to Sally Haslanger, Connie Rosati, Tamar Schapiro, and Brian Slattery. This article originally appeared in a published symposium that also included a commentary on it by Frances Kamm. I had asked the editor for an assurance that there would be no philosophical commentaries, because my article was not originally written for an audience of philosophers. When I received a draft of Kamm's commentary and was asked to respond, I was extremely annoyed at the editor, and I am embarrassed to say that my response vented this annoyance on Kamm instead. I have therefore omitted that response from the present version.

One objection was already clear to me at the time. A few months with cancer had taught me that a tumor rarely invades a region smaller than an extended family.

Physically, the cancer was confined to my body, but even in that respect it was difficult to regard as mine. The tumor cells were growing in my bone marrow, which didn't live up to its poetic billing as the core of my being. The marrow in my bones, I discovered, was as foreign to me as the far side of the moon: it was, in a sense, *my* far side — unseen, insensate — its depth inside me being a measure of remoteness rather than intimacy. Of course, this fertile gunk in my pelvis and skull was also my sole source of blood cells, and my life depended on it. But so did the life of my sons' father, my wife's husband, my parents' son, my brothers' brother, and I was never sure who among us would suffer the greater harm if that life ran out of gunk.

Listening to my host laugh at his future cancer, I wondered whether he realized how many others would share it. What I would have said on their behalf, however, wouldn't have expressed my strongest feelings, which were felt on my own behalf, in a sense that I couldn't articulate. I was somehow offended, insulted. Watching smoke curl from the lips of people unmindful of my mortality, I felt as I probably would feel listening to anti-Semitic remarks directed at another person by a speaker unaware that I, too, was a Jew. I was witnessing an insult to a group of which I was also a member.

This chapter isn't about the right to smoke, of course; it's about the right to die. Not surprisingly, however, these rights tend to be articulated in the same terms. A person claiming either right might describe it, for instance, as a right "to live and die in the light of ... his own convictions about why his life is valuable and where its value lies".

I can't recall whether the speaker in my story used these exact words, but I seemed to hear his voice again when I read them in *The New York Review of Books*, under the title "The Philosophers' Brief".[2] This brief had been submitted to the U.S. Supreme Court in support of a challenge to statutes outlawing physician-assisted suicide. Reading it, I once again felt a collective slight, and this time I couldn't miss which group was being slighted.

---

2   Ronald Dworkin et al., "Assisted Suicide: The Philosophers' Brief", *The New York Review of Books* 44 (March 27, 1997): 41-47. The brief was submitted in the case of *Washington et al. v. Glucksberg et al.*

So I think that I can now explain why I was once offended by one philosopher's defense of smoking, and the explanation leads me to reject The Philosophers' defense of assisted suicide as well. As for assisted suicide itself, however, I don't know what to think. The complexities of the issue have thus far defeated my attempts to arrive at a settled position. On the policy question of assisted suicide, then, I am neither Pro nor Con. I'm, like, Not So Fast.

The principle quoted above, which would settle the issue quickly, can be derived from two broader principles. The first principle is that a person has the right to make his own life shorter in order to make it better — to make it shorter, that is, if doing so is a necessary means or consequence of making it a better life on the whole for him. The second principle is that there is a presumption in favor of deferring to a person's judgment on the subject of his own good. Together, these principles imply that a person has the right to live and die, in particular, by his own convictions about which life would be better for him.

For the smoker in my story, of course, shortening his life was not a means of making it better but rather a likely consequence of an activity that made it better, in his opinion, despite making it shorter, too. But in most of the cases for which assisted suicide is advocated, shortening a patient's life is intended as a means of making it better, because the continuation of the patient's life would detract from its overall value for him.[3] When the first principle is confined to this latter context, it can be rephrased as the assertion of a patient's right to end his life on the grounds that it is no longer worth living.

I think that this principle is mistaken. Before I criticize it, however, I should speak briefly to the second principle stated above, which I can accept. I think that a person's considered judgment about his good is a judgment to which we generally ought to defer.

More specifically, then, I think that we generally ought to defer to a person on the question whether his life is worth living, since the living-worthiness of a life measures the extent to which the continuation of that life would be good for the person living it. The person living a life is the best judge of the value that its continuation would afford him — not an infallible judge, of course, but usually more reliable than anyone else is likely to be.

---

3 I discuss evaluations of this kind in "Well-Being and Time", chapter 7 of this volume.

Indeed, his judgment of this value is to some extent self-fulfilling, since his merely liking or disliking aspects of his life can to some extent make them good or bad for him.

The reasons for deferring to a person's judgment about his good go beyond his reliability as a judge. Respect for a person's autonomy may require that we defer to his considered judgment about his good even when we have reason to regard that judgment as mistaken. Letting him live his own life may sometimes entail letting him make his own mistakes about what's good for him — including, perhaps, mistakes about whether it would be good for him to go on living. Forbidding a person to make such mistakes can be objectionably paternalistic, because it would usurp his role as the primary agent of his own affairs.

Thus, if a person had the right to end his life on the grounds that it wasn't worth living (in accordance with the first principle, above), then he would have the right to be guided by his own judgment on that score (in accordance with the second principle). But I reject the principle that a person has the right to end his life solely on the grounds of the benefits he will thereby obtain or the harms he will avoid.

One reason for rejecting this principle is that a life confers benefits and harms on people other than the person living it. Does a person have the right to deprive his children of a parent simply because life isn't worth enough to him?

I want to set aside this question, however, because it tacitly concedes the assumption that the values at stake in life-or-death decisions are relative to personal interests; it merely invites us to consider a wider circle of potential beneficiaries. The values that we need to consider, in my view, aren't relative to personal interests and consequently have no beneficiaries.

One might insist that values must have beneficiaries, because they wouldn't exist if there weren't someone who could appreciate them: nothing would be good or bad in a universe devoid of sentient beings.[4] But the fact that values wouldn't exist without potential valuers does not entail that they must accrue to someone.

Values are relative to potential valuers because they are normative, in the first instance, for valuation.[5] That is, for something to be valuable just

---

4 See Peter Railton, "Facts and Values", *Philosophical Topics* 14 (1986): 5-31.

5 See Elizabeth Anderson, *Value in Ethics and Economics* (Cambridge, MA: Harvard University Press, 1993).

is for it to be such as ought to be valued in some way — respected, loved, admired, wanted, treasured, or the like. The very concept of value therefore contains the concept of a valuer, actual or potential.

The experience of valuing something can be beneficial, as in the case of appreciating the aesthetic value in a work of art. But the concept of value, in positing a potential valuer, doesn't necessarily require that he would benefit from the experience. Things can be venerable, for example, whether or not there is any benefit in venerating them; and they can be awesome whether or not one would gain by holding them in awe. So the fact that value must be capable of registering with someone, who would thus appreciate it, does not mean that it must be capable of accruing to someone, who would thus gain by it. Value requires a potential valuer but not a potential beneficiary.

In fact, our appreciation of values that are relative to the interest of a beneficiary may depend on a prior appreciation of a value that is not relational in this sense. This dependence emerges when we try to explicate the concept of interest-relative value, or what is good for a person.

The concept of what is good for a person turns out to be fairly resistant to explication. We might initially think to equate what's good for a person with whatever would be rational for him to care about. But this equation would end up implying that all rational concerns are self-interested, by definition. In order to allow for the possibility of rational selflessness, we have to acknowledge that not everything that would be rational for someone to care about is necessarily in his interest.

Various philosophers have therefore attempted to define what's good for a person as a proper subset of the things that would be rational for him to care about, such as the subset including only those things which require his existence. It may or may not be a drawback in these definitions that they would exclude from a person's good such things as posthumous fame. In any case, these definitions are still too inclusive, since the things involving a person's existence that are rational for him to care about include, for example, particular sacrifices that he can make for other people.

The only convincing analysis of a person's good, to my knowledge, is one recently proposed by Stephen Darwall, who argues that what's good for a person is what's rational to want *for his sake*.[6] 'For the sake of' is a phrase that marks the subordination of one concern to another: to care about one thing

---

6   Stephen Darwall, "Self-Interest and Self-Concern", *Social Philosophy and Policy* 14 (1997): 158-178. This article is also the source for my statement of the problem in the preceding section.

for the sake of something else is to care about the former out of concern for the latter. To want something for the sake of a person is thus to want it out of concern for the person himself. Darwall's analysis says that a person's good is what would be rational to want out of concern for that person.

Darwall argues — convincingly, to my mind — that a person's good is a rational object of desire for anyone who cares about that person. By the same token, he argues that even the person himself is rationally obliged to care about his good only insofar as he cares about the person whose good it is — that is, himself.[7]

Think here of the familiar connection between how you feel about yourself and how you feel about your good. Sometimes when you realize that you have done something mean-spirited or shameful, you come to feel worthless as a person; you may even hate yourself; and one symptom of self-hatred is a loss of concern for your own welfare. It no longer seems to matter whether life treats you well or badly, because you yourself seem to be no good. Your desire for your good thus depends on your concern for yourself — and rationally so, according to Darwall's analysis.

Note that self-loathing isn't the feeling that you are worthless *to* yourself. Indeed, the value that things afford to you is precisely what no longer seems to matter, and so your having no value to yourself wouldn't seem to matter, either. The reason why value accruing to you no longer seems to matter, however, is just that *you* don't seem to matter, period. You have lost your appreciation for the value that things have in relation to your interest because you have lost a sense of embodying value in yourself.

Now, things could still be good for you, in Darwall's analysis, even if you didn't embody any value; since they could still be such as *would* be rational for someone to want *if* he cared about you, however baseless the latter concern might be. But things that were good for you would not actually merit concern unless you merited concern; and if you didn't, then despite their being good for you, they wouldn't ultimately be worth wanting, after all. As I put it a moment ago: What's good for you wouldn't matter if you didn't matter.

This account of a person's good therefore implies — rightly, again, in my opinion — that what's good for a person is not a categorical value, any more than what's good for a purpose. What's good for a purpose is worth

---

7 The points made here and in the following paragraph appear in Anderson, *Value in Ethics and Economics*, p. 26.

caring about only out of concern for the purpose, and hence only insofar as the purpose is worth caring about. Similarly, what's good for a person is worth caring about only out of concern for the person, and hence only insofar as he is worth caring about. A person's good has only hypothetical or conditional value, which depends on the value of the person himself.[8]

Of course, we assume that a person's good does matter. But we make this assumption only because we assume that people matter — that everyone has a value that makes him worth caring about. Darwall's analysis of a person's good reveals how our appreciation of value that accrues to someone depends on a prior appreciation of a value inhering in him.

The latter value cannot be relative to personal interests, on pain of setting off a problematic regress. If this value were relative to someone's interest, then it would matter only to the same extent as that beneficiary. This regress of values would continue until it reached a value that was not relative to anyone's interest and that consequently mattered for its own sake. In fact, however, the regress never gets started, because we assume that every person already matters for his own sake, because he embodies an interest-independent value.

A value of this kind, which a person has *in* himself but not *for* anyone, is the basis of Kantian moral theory. Kant's term for this value is 'dignity', and he attributes dignity to all persons in virtue of their rational nature. What morality requires of us, according to Kant, is that we respect the dignity of persons.[9]

The dignity of a person is a value that differs in kind from his interest. Unlike his interest, for example, his dignity is a value on which his opinion carries no more weight than anyone else's. Because this value does not accrue to him, he is in no better position to judge it than others. Similarly, respect for a person's autonomy does not require deference to him on questions of his dignity, as it does on questions of his good. On the contrary, respect for a person's autonomy just is an appreciation of a value in him that amounts to a dignity, in Kant's sense of the term, precisely because

---

8 This point, too, is made by Anderson.

9 Here I am making a leap that requires more justification than I can provide in the present context. I am equating the value that we appreciate in caring about a person with the value that we appreciate, somewhat differently, in respecting that person in the Kantian sense. I defend this equation in "Love as a Moral Emotion", *Ethics* 109 (1999): 338-374, reprinted in *Self to Self: Selected Essays* (New York: Cambridge University Press, 2005), pp. 70-109.

it commands respect. If a person denies embodying such a value, he can hardly claim that we should defer to him out of an appreciation for a value such as he denies. He cannot claim, in other words, that out of respect for his autonomy we should defer to his judgment that he possesses nothing worthy of our respect.

Nor is it paternalistic to challenge a person's judgment about his dignity, as it is in the case of his good. Challenging a person's judgment about his good is objectionable because it undermines his role as the agent of his own affairs; but his value as a person is not just his affair. Although his good is a value that accrues to him alone, in the first instance, his value as a person inheres in him among other persons. It's a value that he possesses by virtue of being one of us, and the value of being one of us is not his alone to assess or defend. The value of being a person is therefore something larger than any particular person who embodies it.

That's what I miss in so many discussions of euthanasia and assisted suicide: a sense of something in each of us that is larger than any of us, something that makes human life more than just an exchange of costs for benefits, more than just a job or a trip to the mall. I miss the sense of a value in us that makes a claim on us — a value that we must *live up to*.

I don't deny that there are circumstances under which it would be better for one's life to end and permissible to hasten its ending. What I deny is that one may end one's life simply because one isn't getting enough *out* of it. One has to consider whether one is doing justice *to* it.

If a person possesses no value that he must live up to, or do justice to, then his life becomes a mere instrument, to be used or discarded according to whether it serves his interest. His moral claim to his own life then looks something like this:

> [A] patient's right to life includes a right not to be killed. But that right gives [him] a protected option whether to live or die, an option with which others cannot legitimately interfere; it does not give [him] a duty to live. If a patient decides to die, he is waiving his right to live. By waiving his right, he releases others (perhaps a specific other person) from a duty not to kill him.

This can't be right. It portrays morality as protecting a person's options without protecting the person himself, except insofar as his own existence is one of his options. Surely, however, options are worth protecting, not for their own sake, but for the sake of the person whose options they are. So how can morality treat the person as worth protecting only for the sake of protecting one of his options? If he doesn't already merit protection, how can they?

The quotation above is drawn from an essay by Frances Kamm, who goes on to answer Kantian objections as follows:[10]

> Suppose life involves such unbearable pain that one's whole life is focused on that pain. In such circumstances, one could, I believe, decline the honor of being a person. …We might acknowledge the great (and normally overriding) value of being a person … [and yet] allow that some bad conditions may overshadow its very great value.

Here Kamm is claiming that someone can view life as a mere option even while accepting the Kantian view of his value as a person. The problem with this passage is that it misstates the Kantian view.

When Kamm says that the value of a person normally "overrid[es]" the value of other goods, but can be "overshadow[ed]" by conditions that are exceptionally bad, she implies that it can be balanced against the person's interest. And when she goes on to speak of this value as an "honor" that the person can decline, she implies that it is actually part of a person's interest, since an honor accrues to a particular person, whose role as its beneficiary entitles him to accept or decline it.

But the dignity of a person isn't something that he can accept or decline, since it isn't a value *for* him; it's a value *in* him, which he can only violate or respect. Nor can it be weighed against what is good or bad for the person. As I have argued, value *for* a person stands to value *in* the person roughly as the value of means stands to that of the end: in each case, the former merits concern only on the basis of concern for the latter. And conditional values cannot be weighed against the unconditional values on which they depend. The value of means to an end cannot overshadow or be overshadowed by the value of the end, because it already is only a shadow of that value, in the sense of being dependent upon it. Similarly, the value of what's good for a person is only a shadow of the value inhering in the person, and cannot overshadow or be overshadowed by it.

---

10 Frances Kamm, "A Right to Choose Death?", *Boston Review* 22 (1997): 20-23.

These are abstract considerations, but they are concretely illustrated by the story with which I began. When my host claimed that he benefited more from the pleasures of smoking than he would be harmed by an early death, my first thought was that he had failed to consider harms and benefits to people other than himself. On second thought, however, I resented his assumption that harms and benefits were the only values at stake.

My host's remarks implied that an early death, of the sort he was risking and I was hoping to forestall, would be a loss to him that could be offset by sufficient gains. But what would it matter how much I lost or gained if I myself would be no loss? My gains or losses would merit concern only on the basis of concern for me — which, being the basis of concern for them, could not then be offset by that concern. Hence, my gains or losses wouldn't matter unless I had a value that could not be offset by theirs.

My host was implicitly denying the existence of such a value. For he claimed that death was worth worrying about only in respects for which he could be compensated by the pleasures of smoking. He was thus implicitly denying the interest-independent value of a person, without which it couldn't really matter whether I lived or died.

Of course, he was denying the existence of this value in his own case, not in mine; but our cases were indistinguishable on this score. By implicitly denying his own interest-independent value, my host was somehow trivializing or denigrating himself as a person. Sometimes people's self-denigrating remarks just embarrass us, but in other instances they can be sufficiently principled to give offense. Recall my earlier reference to anti-Semitism. Anti-Semitism can manifest itself in self-denigrating remarks, if it is the anti-Semitism of a self-hating Jew. My host's disregard for his own value as a person offended me as another person, just as someone's denigrating himself as a Jew would offend me as another Jew.

I think Kant was right to say that trading one's person in exchange for benefits, or relief from harms, denigrates the value of personhood, respect for which is a criterion of morality (Kant would say, *the* criterion). That's why I think that smoking is a vice — at least, when practiced for the reasons offered by my host. It's also why I think that suicide is immoral when committed on the grounds that life isn't worth living.

Mind you, I don't go around snatching cigarettes out of people's mouths. And I'm not sure that I would forcibly try to stop someone from committing suicide solely because it would be immorally self-destructive. The impermissibility of someone else's conduct doesn't necessarily give me permission to interfere with it. By the same token, however, I think that encouraging or assisting others in impermissible conduct is itself impermissible. That's why I think that the tobacco industry is engaged in an immoral enterprise. And it's why I think the same of Dr. Kevorkian, who has done more than anyone to help people die by their own convictions.

Note that these moral judgments distinguish between self-destruction and mere self-harm. As I have said, I believe that people are sometimes entitled to act on mistaken judgments about their own interest; and to this extent, at least, they are entitled to harm themselves. But the behaviors that I have criticized don't merely damage the agents' interests; indeed, they may not damage the agents' interests at all, if the agents are right about the costs and benefits involved. These behaviors are to be criticized, in my view, because they are premised on a disregard for the value of the agents themselves.

The same criticism would apply, for example, to agents who put up their own freedom as collateral in order to obtain loans. People have no right to sell themselves into slavery, no matter what their convictions, but the reason is not that they would thereby be harming themselves; the reason is that they would be violating their own personhood.

These moral judgments depend, of course, on my belief that a person has an interest-independent value; and they may consequently seem to impose my Kantian values even on people who don't believe in them. Don't people have the right to live and die by their own convictions as to the value of their lives?

If the question is whether people are morally permitted to end their existence solely because they find it unrewarding, then I have already answered in the negative, on the grounds that they would then be violating their own interest-independent value as persons. But of course the present question is meant to be taken differently, as suggesting that we defer to people's judgments about whether they have an interest-independent value, in the first place. Under this interpretation, the question is not whether people are permitted to violate their own dignity but whether they are entitled to be believed when they insist that they have none. I have answered in the negative to this latter version of the question as well. The reasons for deferring to people about values relative to their interests do not apply in the case of interest-independent value.

This answer may seem to beg the question, since it presupposes the existence of the very interest-independent value that is at issue. What I have now argued, however, is that we cannot avoid presupposing the existence of this value anyway, since it's needed to account for the importance of interest-relative values. We cannot justify someone's death on the grounds that it's good for him, while also denying the existence of another value, embodied in him. For if he were himself a cipher, evaluatively speaking, then what's good for him would be, in the same manner of speaking, good for nothing.

I admit that talk of someone's value as a person sounds like religion rather than philosophy. Such talk is a secular version of religious talk about the sanctity of human life.

Historically speaking, however, most moral discourse has religious sources. The question for secular ethics is whether we can rationally accept the values bequeathed to us by religion while being skeptical of their theological basis. A question that's equally pressing, though less widely acknowledged, is whether we can selectively accept some of these values while discarding others. My view is that our values will be incoherent so long as they lack a counterpart to the sanctity of human life.

This view will immediately seem to entail reactionary consequences, such as a rejection of euthanasia and abortion in any form. But a secular value that corresponds to the sanctity of human life needn't be exactly the same value or yield exactly the same consequences. In particular, it need not attach to biological life or biological humanity per se; and so it needn't rule out abortion, for example, simply because the fetus is both alive and human. What secular morality must regard as sacrosanct, I have suggested, is not the human organism but the person, and a fetus may embody one but not the other.

Recognizing the interest-independent value of a person wouldn't necessarily rule out euthanasia or suicide, either. On the contrary, recognizing such a value is essential to one familiar argument in favor of these practices — namely, the argument for dying with dignity.

The idea that dignity can justify a person's death may seem incompatible with the Kantian conception of dignity as a value inhering in the person. Wouldn't a person's value always militate in favor of saving his life?

This apparent conflict is due, however, to a confusion about the normative implications of dignity. Dignity is what Kant called a "self-existent" value — a value to which we are obliged to respond only when it already exists, and then only by paying it reverence or respect. The value of persons does not oblige us to maximize the number of people in existence; it obliges us only to respect the people who do exist. And respecting these people is not necessarily a matter of keeping them in existence; it is rather a matter of treating them in the way that is required by their personhood — whatever way that is.[11]

The Kantian objection to suicide, then, is not that it destroys something of value. The objection is not even to suicide per se, but to suicide committed for a particular kind of reason — that is, in order to obtain benefits or escape harms. And the objection to suicide committed for this reason is that it denigrates the person's dignity, by trading his person for interest-relative goods, as if it were one of them. This interpretation of the objection to suicide leaves open the possibility that a person's dignity may justify suicide in other contexts, if suicide would constitute an appropriate expression of respect for one's person. Kantianism would then be able to endorse the notion of dying with dignity.[12]

Actually, the phrase 'dying with dignity' is potentially misleading. We don't think that a person's death is morally acceptable so long as he can carry it off with dignity. Rather, we think that a person's death is acceptable if he can no longer live with dignity. The operative concept is undignified life, not dignified death.

When a person cannot sustain both life and dignity, his death may indeed be morally justified. One is sometimes permitted, even obligated, to destroy objects of dignity if they would otherwise deteriorate in ways that would offend against that value. The moral obligation to bury or burn a corpse, for example, is an obligation not to let it become an affront to what it once was. Librarians have similar practices for destroying tattered books — and honor guards, for destroying tattered flags — out of respect for the dignity inherent in these objects.

---

11 The interpretation of Kant expressed in this paragraph is not uncontroversial. I defend it at length in "Love as a Moral Emotion".

12 For a Kantian argument along these lines, see Thomas E. Hill, Jr., "Self-Regarding Suicide: A Modified Kantian View", in his *Autonomy and Self-Respect* (Cambridge: Cambridge University Press, 1991), pp. 85-103.

Of course, the value inhering in mere things, such as books or flags, must be different from that inhering in persons by virtue of their rational nature. But all of these values belong together as a class, the class of dignity values, whose defining characteristic is that they call for reverence or respect.[13]

These examples suggest that dignity can require not only the preservation of what possesses it but also the destruction of what is losing it, if the loss would be irretrievable.[14] Dignity, unlike well-being, does not come in degrees that we are obliged to maximize; as we have seen, it is not a value whose existence we are obliged to promote at all. To treat a dignity value as capable of degrees, all of them worth preserving, would be to treat it like an ordinary good — which would in fact be disrespectful. Respect for an object of dignity can sometimes require its destruction.

The question, then, is what constitutes the loss of dignity for a person. The dignity in question has nothing to do with being dignified, with keeping up appearances, or with sustaining any particular social status. It has nothing to do with what people ought to admire or esteem in one another, or with what they actually respect. It is rather what they ought to respect, in the way that they can manifest only by treating one another morally. According to Kant, what people ought to respect in this way is one another's rational nature.

Ironically, Kant's view is borne out by Kamm's example, in which "life involves such unbearable pain that one's whole life is focused on that pain". Kamm assumes that this case invites us to weigh the disvalue of pain against the value of being a rational agent. In fact, however, Kamm has described a case in which pain is more than painful, since it not only hurts the patient but also becomes the sole focus of his life. Pain that tyrannizes the patient in this fashion undermines his rational agency, by preventing

---

13 Actually, I am inclined to think that the dignity of books or flags is borrowed from the dignity of personhood; but this question is beyond the scope of the present chapter.

14 I believe that this feature of dignity values explains why the permissibility of euthanasia and assisted suicide is limited mainly to cases of terminal illness. Felicia Ackerman has claimed that such a restricted permission is unstable ("Assisted Suicide, Terminal Illness, Severe Disability, and the Double Standard", in *Physician-Assisted Suicide: Expanding the Debate*, ed. Margaret P. Battin, Rosamond Rhodes, and Anita Silvers [New York: Routledge, 1998], pp. 149-161). She argues that assistance in dying must be permissible either for all competent adults or for none. I agree with Ackerman that the arguments usually offered in favor of assistance in dying cannot be restricted to cases of terminal illness, although their proponents often adopt that restriction anyway, without justification. As Ackerman shows, e.g., the arguments of "The Philosophers' Brief" support assisted suicide for everyone if they support it for anyone. But I think that the Kantian view can justify the restriction and that its ability to do so counts in its favor.

him from choosing any ends for himself other than relief. It reduces the patient to the psychological hedonist's image of a person — a pleasure-seeking, pain-fleeing animal — which is undignified indeed. And Kamm is clearly envisioning that this severely reduced condition of the patient can be ended only by his death.

I suspect, then, that if euthanasia seems justified in Kamm's example, the reason is not that relieving the patient's pain is more important than his dignity as a person; the reason is rather that pain has already undermined the patient's dignity, and irretrievably so. The example thus supports dying for the sake of dignity, not for the sake of self- interest.

I often wonder whether proponents of assisted suicide don't overstate the moral significance of pain. Pain is a bad thing, of course, but I doubt whether it can justify anything close to euthanasia or suicide unless it is (as Kamm calls it) unbearable. And then what justifies death is the unbearableness of the pain rather than the painfulness.

What do we mean in calling pain unbearable? What is it *not to bear* pain? It certainly isn't a matter of refusing to feel the pain, of shutting one's eyes to it, as one might to an unbearable sight, or of walking away from it, as one might from an unbearable situation. Not to bear pain is somehow to fall apart in the face of it, to disintegrate as a person. To find pain unbearable is to find it thus destructive not just of one's well-being but of oneself.

But then we make a mistake if we describe the patient in unbearable pain as if he were his rational old self, weighing the harm of pain against the benefits of existence. If his pain is truly unbearable, then he isn't his rational self any longer: he is falling apart in pain. Even if he enjoys some moments of relief and clarity, he is still falling apart diachronically, a temporally scattered person at best.

I don't think that we serve the patient well in these circumstances by claiming broad rights of self-determination in his name. He may indeed be entitled to help in dying, and he will certainly have to participate in the relevant decisions. But let us keep in mind that these decisions would be premature if the patient were not already in the twilight of his autonomy, where self-determination is more of a shadowy presumption than a clear fact.

I do not know how to frame a public policy or law that would distinguish between the cases in which I think that euthanasia or suicide is morally permissible and the cases in which I think it is not. Of course, the law would not have to follow the moral vicissitudes of the practice so closely if they were covered by a right of self-determination. If there were a broad class of cases in which the patient had the right to decide for himself whether death was justified, then we could legalize euthanasia or assisted suicide in those cases, even though it might not be justified in all of them. If a patient then opted for death when it wasn't justified, he would still be acting within his rights, which the law would have been justified in protecting.

But I do not believe that a person has the right, in general, to choose between life and death; nor do I believe that a person's rights suddenly expand when he becomes terminally ill. So I don't see how a case for legalization can be founded on rights of self-determination, and I am once again faced with the difficulty of legalizing death for the sake of dignity without also legalizing it for the sake of self-interest.

I certainly don't think that the law should forbid activities simply because they have the potential of being self-destructive in some circumstances. I don't think that mountain climbing should be outlawed — or smoking, for that matter. The problem is that killing, unlike mountain climbing or smoking, impinges on the dignity of persons essentially and not just in some unfortunate circumstances or cases. The result is that the law on killing, like the law on slavery, unavoidably expresses our collective valuation of personhood itself.

Supporters of euthanasia and assisted suicide sometimes liken them to the other intrinsically injurious treatments to which a patient may consent for his greater good — the cutting and stabbing and drugging and poisoning that are the physician's stock in trade. Then they ask: What's so special about killing?[15] Isn't killing just another medical intervention to which a patient should be allowed to submit when it serves his interest? My inclination is to answer this question with another: What's so special about slavery? Isn't enslavement just another cost that a person should be allowed to risk in pursuit of his interests?

Surely, there is something special about slavery. Though we may indeed have a right to live and die in light of our own convictions, it doesn't extend to convictions about the price for which our freedom would be worth selling. Nor does it extend, in my view, to convictions about the price for which our lives would be worth ending. And self-interested reasons for

---

15 Kamm asks this question in section 4 of "A Right to Choose Death?"

ending our lives are, in the Kantian sense, reasons of price rather than dignity.

When it comes to the design of public policy on assisted suicide, I am inclined to think that considerations about the morality of the practice itself may be swamped by considerations about the collateral effects of legalization. As I have argued elsewhere, simply allowing people to opt for death may eliminate the conditions that make some people's lives worth living, thereby creating new candidates for killing.[16] Legalization would therefore do harm to people who are currently no more than bystanders to the debate.

These collateral harms might have to be tolerated if there were a fundamental right to choose between life and death. We can't deprive all people of a choice to which they're morally entitled just because some people would be better off without it.

What I have argued here, however, is that there isn't a fundamental right to choose between life and death. There may still be a moral justification for death in some cases, but it doesn't rest on a right of self-determination. And without such a right, the case for legalization must proceed more slowly — far more slowly than The Philosophers would like us to believe.

---

16 See "Against the Right to Die", chapter 2 of this volume.

4. Beyond Price[1]

Kant argued that suicide is immoral when committed for the purpose of escaping from unhappiness. I have tried on one or two occasions to reconstruct Kant's argument, by offering a particular interpretation of the Formula of Humanity, which says that a person has a value that makes him an end in himself.[2] The statement that a person is an end, I interpret as expressing the fact that we ought to care about some things for the person's sake, by caring about them out of concern for him. A person is an end in the sense that he is that for the sake of which — out of concern for which — some things are worth caring about. This conception of how a person can be an end yields an argument against escapist suicide, I argued, when it is combined with a particular conception of a person's good, which is what the escapist attempts to serve by cutting his life short.

I borrowed the latter conception from Stephen Darwall, who contends that a person's good consists in what it would be rational to care about for the person's sake in the sense of caring about it out of concern for the

1   This chapter is a substantially revised version of a paper that appeared in *Ethics* 118 (2008): 191-212, http://dx.doi.org/10.1086/523746. The first version of the paper was presented to a workshop on value at Columbia University. I am grateful to the participants for helpful discussion: Ruth Chang, Jonathan Dancy, Jim Griffin, Ulrike Heuer, Tom Hurka, Shelly Kagan, Frances Kamm, Maggie Little, Véronique Munoz-Dardé, Peter Railton, Joseph Raz, Jacob Ross, Michael Smith, and Larry Temkin. A subsequent version was presented to the philosophy department at the University of Miami and to the Legal Theory Workshop at Yale Law School. Thanks to Shelly Kagan and Ruth Marcus for additional comments on the latter occasion. Finally, it was presented to a conference organized by Jeanette Kennett at the Centre for Applied Philosophy and Public Ethics of the Australian National University.
2   "A Right of Self-Termination?", chapter 3 of this volume; "A Brief Introduction to Kantian Ethics", in *Self to Self: Selected Essays* (New York: Cambridge University Press, 2005), pp. 16-44; and "Reading Kant's *Groundwork*", in *Ethics: Essential Readings in Moral Theory*, ed. George Sher (New York: Routledge, 2012), pp. 343-359.

person.[3] Since this structure of concerns is the one that explains how a person can be an end, in my view, I suggested that a person's good stands to the value of a person in a relation analogous to (though of course distinct from) that of means to an ordinary end, the former member of either pair being worth caring about for the sake of, or out of concern for, the latter. I then argued that escapist suicide entails a practical irrationality analogous to that of sacrificing an end for the sake of the means to it.

Such an irrationality is committed, for example, by people who grub for money. Money has value only as a means to happiness (let's assume), but money-grubbers make themselves unhappy in the pursuit of money, thereby sacrificing happiness for the sake of something that is valuable only for its sake. A person makes a similar mistake, I argued, if he sacrifices himself for the sake of something that is valuable only for his sake by committing suicide to promote his own good. In either case, one thing (money, an end to unhappiness) is preferred to another (happiness, the person himself) even though it is worth caring about only out of concern for that to which it is preferred.

This analogy is open to two objections. Let me start with the one that I know how to answer.

The answerable objection goes like this. The reason why money is valuable for the sake of happiness is that it is instrumental to producing happiness, but the reason why relieving someone's unhappiness is valuable for his sake is not that it's instrumental to producing *him*. So whereas destroying happiness defeats the purpose of money, destroying oneself doesn't clearly defeat the purpose of ending one's unhappiness. Ending one's unhappiness is good for oneself in a sense that doesn't entail its having a purpose at all: its ultimate end is not a purpose but a person. What, then, is there to be defeated?[4]

---

3   Stephen Darwall, *Welfare and Rational Care* (Princeton, NJ: Princeton University Press, 2004).

4   Objections to my argument were first raised by Frances Kamm in "Physician-Assisted Suicide, the Doctrine of Double Effect, and the Ground of Value", *Ethics* 109 (1999): 586-605. I am now dissatisfied with the responses I made to Kamm in my appendix to "A Right of Self-Termination?", which I have omitted from the version reprinted as chapter 3 of this volume. I was prompted to revisit this debate by a discussion of the latter article at the Colloquium on Legal, Political, and Social Philosophy at New York University (led by Thomas Nagel and Ronald Dworkin), especially by Nagel's comments on that occasion.

The answer to this objection is that it misinterprets the analogy between a person and an ordinary end. Of course there is no instrumental relation between ending a person's unhappiness and the person himself, but the instrumental relation between money and happiness is not what makes grubbing for money irrational anyway. What makes it irrational to seek money at the cost of happiness is that money is worth wanting only out of a desire for happiness. Seeking money at the cost of happiness thwarts the desire out of which money is worth caring about to begin with. The instrumental relation of money to happiness explains why the one is worth caring about out of concern for the other, but the irrationality in the case is generated by the resulting relation between these concerns, one of which depends on the other but is served in such a way as to frustrate it: the desire for money is served in such a way as to frustrate the desire for happiness, on which it depends. A similar relation obtains between ending one's unhappiness through suicide and the value of the person himself: the one is worth caring about only out of concern for the other. A similar irrationality will be generated, then, if killing oneself thwarts the concern out of which ending one's unhappiness is worth caring about, to begin with.

But now comes the second objection, which is not so easily answered: How does killing oneself thwart the concern out of which ending one's unhappiness is worth caring about? An end to one's unhappiness is worth caring about, I claim, out of concern for one's value as a person. But how is that latter concern frustrated when one pursues an end to unhappiness by means of suicide? This question becomes especially pressing in light of Kant's view about a person's value and its proper mode of appreciation. According to Kant, a person is a self-existent end, which is to be valued as it is, given that it exists, rather than as a thing to be brought into existence. And the mode of appreciation proper to such an end is respect, which is an attitude of self-restraint, inhibiting us from violating the person's autonomy.

Well, killing a person does seem to violate his autonomy, to say the least. But when the victim is also the killer, his killing may be an exercise of his autonomy, too — so how can it qualify as a violation? Maybe escapist suicide, at worst, is a case of autonomy violating itself, a case toward which the attitude of respect must be, at worst, ambivalent. In that case, suicide would not exactly thwart the concern that underlies its own motivation.[5]

---

5   I am tempted to reply that escapist suicide is not autonomous, precisely because it is irrational. But I am trying to demonstrate its irrationality on the grounds that it thwarts the concern underlying its own motivation; if that concern is respect for autonomy, then

Surely, though, the argument was already in trouble once respect for autonomy was introduced. Respect was introduced in the role of that appreciation for a person's value out of which it makes sense to care about the person's good. But respect is simply the wrong attitude for that role. Rather than sort out whether suicide is more expressive than destructive of autonomy, let us consider alternative attitudes to which the motive for escapist suicide might more plausibly be subordinate.

Darwall proposes that the response out of which things are worth valuing when they are valuable for a person's sake, is an attitude that he calls "sympathetic concern" for that person. This proposal will be vacuous, of course, if sympathetic concern must be defined as a concern for the person's interests: to define a person's interests as comprising whatever is worth valuing out of concern for his interests would be tautologous. But Darwall argues that sympathetic concern can be identified without being defined, since it is a natural kind of affective response, which can be singled out by paradigm instances.

Yet I suspect that sympathy, like respect, is ill-suited to serve as the concern in relation to which a person's interests should be defined. Although sympathy is not the same as empathy, it is an empathic response — a variant of empathy — and so it focuses on the feelings of its object. What sympathetic concern for a person disposes us to care about will therefore tend to be the state of his feelings, and the resulting conception of a person's good must consequently have a bias toward hedonism. While I don't think that the very concept of a person's good should rule out hedonism, I don't think that it should rule in its favor, either.

Moreover, what would make sense to care about out of sympathetic concern for a person is not necessarily what we would judge to be in that person's interest. For example, parents who think that the welfare of their child requires them to administer punishment or harsh medicine may be inhibited from doing so precisely by sympathetic concern. In order to do what's best for the child, they may have to overcome their sympathetic impulses — which suggests that sympathy is not always a reliable guide to the well-being of its object.[6]

I am at risk of arguing in a circle. For if escapist suicide is irrational because it thwarts respect for autonomy, and it thwarts that concern because it isn't autonomous, then the reason why it isn't autonomous cannot be that it is irrational.

6   Of course, one might argue that punishing the child would express a higher or better-informed sympathy than sparing the child. But such an argument would seem to rely on a prior conception of the child's interests, as a basis for privileging one form of sympathy

Suppose that the parent punishes the child, saying, "I'm doing this for your own good." The parent would be unlikely to elaborate by saying, "So, you see, I'm doing it out of sympathy for you." They both know that insofar as he feels sympathy, the parent is acting in spite of it. If he offers any elaboration on the claim to be acting for the child's good, he is more likely to say, "So, you see, I'm doing this because I love you." Thus, if the child's good is that which is worth caring about out of some attitude toward the child, then the relevant attitude is not sympathy but love.[7]

Maybe this emendation to Darwall's conception of well-being can yield an emendation to the argument that I rested upon it — my argument for a rational obstacle to escapist suicide. Fashioning such an emendation will be my aim in the rest of this chapter.

If a person's good is to be analyzed as that which is worth caring about out of love for the person, then the relevant form of love must be carefully distinguished from the romantic or sexual emotion that goes by the same name — the love of falling or being "in" love — since romantic or sexual love is largely possessive, even self-seeking. The same goes for various other attitudes that tend to accompany love, such as attachment. We can feel attached to people without loving them, and we can love people to whom we are not especially attached.

There is a sense of the verb 'to love' that denotes a kind of solicitous behavior that characterizes the familial relationships with which the emotion is conventionally associated. The "loving mother" or "loving husband" of standard obituaries was loving in this sense — actively attentive, affectionate, caring. Many philosophers assume that the emotion of love must be the attitude that naturally motivates such behavior, hence a benevolent form of affection. There certainly is such an attitude, and there is nothing wrong with calling it "love".

Yet benevolent affection is an emotion that we can recognize animals as manifesting toward their young; it is also felt by children for their special toys, by gardeners for their flowers, and by philatelists for their stamps. This emotion is unlikely to reveal anything that we don't already know

---

as higher or better-informed than another; so it seems to reverse the order of analysis in Darwall's account, by identifying the relevant valuing attitude in terms of well-being rather than vice versa.

7 The following discussion of love is an attempt to summarize and expand upon my discussion in "Love as a Moral Emotion", *Ethics* 109 (1999): 338-374, reprinted in *Self to Self*, pp. 70-109.

about the interests of these beloved objects. The *philia* of philately is not, I think, an emotion whose nature will help us to understand what is best for stamps. The philatelist does indeed take loving care of his stamps, but he does so under the guidance of some antecedent conception of what it is for stamps to be in good condition. He cannot simply love his stamps and let his heart be his guide.

Yet there is an emotion, also called love, which is indeed a guide to the interests of the beloved. This emotion is present in many loving relationships, where it can be difficult to disentangle from benevolent affection, but it can be absent from such relationships as well. People can take loving care of companions or wards with genuine feeling that nevertheless amounts to no more than fondness, because it falls short of that fiercer emotion that can only be called love. Conversely, they can feel the latter emotion for someone without being thereby moved to treat him lovingly, as becomes especially clear in relationships carried on at arm's length. Students can love a teacher — or patients, a doctor — without having any inclination to cuddle or coddle him; there can be love between colleagues who would never presume to take care of one another; and even loving friendships can be characterized by a formality that rules out intrusions into one another's lives. Finally, what I have described as the fiercer and more compelling form of love can coexist with, can indeed give rise to, the very opposite of benevolent affection, in the form of hostility or even hate. You can want to hurt someone you love, and both your love for him and your desire to hurt him can still be wholehearted.

This last possibility is not incompatible with my suggestion that love is a guide to the interests of the beloved. The suggestion is not that love necessarily involves a desire for the good of the beloved or — to correct the order of analysis — that a person's good is that which loving him would necessarily involve a desire for. Rather, the suggestion modifies Darwall's account by saying that a person's good is that which is worth caring about, or which makes sense to care about, out of love for that person. And the acknowledgment that love needn't involve a desire for the beloved's good is perfectly compatible with the claim that it provides a natural motive or reason for such a desire. Or — to correct the order of analysis once again — the acknowledgment that what is wanted by a lover need not be good for the beloved is compatible with the claim that what is worth wanting, or makes sense to want, out of love for the person is indeed what is good for him.

The question is what love makes it appropriate or rational to care about. More specifically, the question is what can constitute a person's good by virtue of being that which loving him makes it appropriate or rational to care about — a question to which the answer must be more substantive than "the person's good". Here I want to adopt a suggestion from Connie Rosati, who has criticized Darwall's sympathy-based account of well-being as follows:[8] "When we appreciate the value, as it seems to us, of a work of art, we endeavor to preserve it in its valuable condition. Likewise, when we appreciate, as it seems to us, the value of a person, we seek to preserve the person in her condition as the valuable being she is. Just what attitude might capture this idea without itself involving concern for a person's welfare, I will not venture to guess. But care or sympathetic concern seems not to be it."

Clearly, loving someone is a way of appreciating his value. Rosati's analogy therefore suggests that what it makes sense to care about out of love for a person is the preservation of the value or the valuable condition to which love is an appreciative response.

The next question, of course, is what sort of value or valuable condition is appreciated by love. Some philosophers would understand this question as equivalent to the question what we love people for; and they would answer it by citing the various qualities for which we love our parents, spouses, children, and friends — their fine characters, their fetching looks, their sense of humor, or their shared history with us. But I have difficulty believing that the value to which we respond in loving people is conferred on them by the miscellaneous qualities that we profess to love them for. As many philosophers have pointed out, we often profess to love people even for their flaws; but surely loving them doesn't give us reason for wanting those flaws to be perpetuated.

My view is that loving a person "for" some quality is not a matter of responding to a value conferred on him by that quality.[9] Rather, I claim, the

---

8   Connie S. Rosati, "Darwall on Welfare and Rational Care", *Philosophical Studies* 30 (2006): 619-635, p. 626.

9   Of course, we can love someone without there being anything for which we love him. See D. W. Hamlyn, "The Phenomena of Love and Hate", *Philosophy* 53 (1978): 5-20, p. 8: "To be loved full-stop is simply to be loved without there being anything that the love is for. In such a situation there is likely to be some explanation why the love came into being,

qualities for which we love someone are qualities that show us or remind us or symbolize for us that value to which we respond by loving him. They are signs of his value, not its substance. To find someone's crooked smile endearing is not to find him more valuable in virtue of smiling crookedly; it is rather to find the smile emblematic of what is valuable about him, which would still be valuable even if his smile were straight.

The value that makes people proper objects of love is a topic that seems to be surrounded by paradox. In loving someone, we treasure him as special and irreplaceable; yet we love more than one person, and we believe that almost everyone is worthy of being loved by someone. If everyone is worthy of being loved, however, then everyone is worthy of being treasured as special, and so everyone must *be* special — in which case, there must be nothing special, or at least nothing especially special, about anyone. There's a paradox for you. Here is another. We love our own children above all other children, and yet we don't honestly believe that our children are more valuable than others. How can we be so selective in appreciating a value that we acknowledge to be virtually universal?

Niko Kolodny has argued that our reasons for loving a person lie in our relationship with the person — his being our parent, spouse, child, or friend. What makes someone special, according to this view, is that he is special *to us* by virtue of sharing a particular relationship *with* us. Everyone can be special, then, because everyone can be special to someone, with whom he shares a similar relationship.

Although I find much to admire in Kolodny's discussion of love, I find his thesis unpersuasive. We probably cannot love people with whom we aren't acquainted, but I think that we can indeed love acquaintances with whom we have no significant relationship — love them at first sight or from afar. We can also love people whose relationship with us we do not value at all, as when divorcing couples still love one another despite looking back on their marriage as a disaster from day one. People who are estranged from their parents or siblings generally say that refusing to have any further dealings with these people does not entail loving them any less.[10]

---

and it is possible with some objects of love for one to love them for the fact that and because of the circumstances in which the love came into being; but there seems to me no necessity that it should be like that — the circumstances may explain the continuance of the love but they may not be what the love is for. I suggest that love is possible where there is nothing that the love is for."

10 See Hamlyn, "The Phenomena of Love and Hate", p. 9: "It might be [said] that it must at least be true that the lover desires the beloved, wants to be with him/her/it, or something

At a more fundamental level, I find love as Kolodny conceives it to be self-centered, since it responds to a value that the beloved has, not because of what he is in himself, but because of what he is to us. Love so conceived is a response to a fundamentally egocentric value, a value that others have in virtue of the part they play in our lives. I doubt whether love is really so egocentric.

In responding to a related objection, Kolodny says: [11]

> Nevertheless, it may be replied, even if we are not valued only instrumentally on the relationship theory, we are still valued extrinsically and nonfinally. Our relatives value us, it might be said, in the way one might value a now useless pen that once belonged to Winston Churchill: as an [intrinsically] worthless object that merits a certain response only because it is associated with something of final worth. This analogy, however, is misleading in at least two respects. First, our relatives do not deny that we are finally valuable. However else they view us, they view us as persons, and hence as beings with final value. Second, it is not the case that our relatives' valuing us is optional, given that they value their relationships to us. According to the relationship theory, their valuing us is constitutive of their valuing their relationships to us, in the sense that they cannot respond appropriately to the value of their relationships to us without also valuing us. Admiring Churchill, by contrast, does not require fetishizing his possessions.

Here Kolodny concedes that when people love us, they regard us as valuable in ourselves, because they regard *us* as persons. Yet according to Kolodny, this appreciation of our value as persons is distinct from people's love for us, which is based instead on our relationship with them.

In my view, appreciation for someone's value as a person is not distinct from loving him: it is the evaluative core of love. I do not mean that love is a value judgment to the effect that the beloved has final value as an end in himself. Love is rather an appreciative response to the perception of that value. And I mean "perception" literally: the people we love are the ones whom we succeed in *perceiving* as persons within some of the human organisms milling about us. Only sometimes in this throng do we vividly see a face or hear a voice or feel a touch as animated by the inner presence

---

of that kind. I am not sure that even this has to be true. Suppose that someone has got to the point of recognizing the absolutely disastrous character of a relationship. It is possible for them to renounce it and any desire for its continuance while still loving the person concerned."

11 Niko Kolodny, "Love as Valuing a Relationship", *The Philosophical Review* 112 (2003): 135-189, p. 156. I have substituted the word 'intrinsically' for 'extrinsically' in the original passage, on the assumption that the latter is a misprint.

of a self-aware, autonomous other — a person who is self to himself, like us. Iris Murdoch says that "love is the extremely difficult realisation that something other than oneself is real"[12] — that some*one* other than oneself is real, I would say, in the case of love for a person. A sense of wonder at the vividly perceived reality of another person is, in my view, the essence of love.

It is because the reality of other persons is not directly perceptible to us that we love people for their faces and voices — and even their flaws — which somehow alert us to the presence of another inner life alongside our own. Not every smile strikes us quite forcibly with the presence of the person behind it — not one in a million — which is why we love but one in a million, perhaps for his smile. We do not see most people for what they are, even if we know what they are. And what *are* they, that they are worthy of being loved, except other persons like ourselves?

This explanation for the selectivity of love still doesn't solve the puzzle of everyone's being worthy of love and hence worthy of being valued as special. Even if each of us can value only a few people as special, the thought that everyone deserves to be so valued seems to imply that everyone actually is special — in which case, no one is special, after all.

The solution to this puzzle, I think, is to realize that what makes a person special is not a value that sets him apart from others; it's a value that calls for appreciating him by setting him apart, a mode of appreciation that considers him alone. The key to this solution is that values are normative, in the first instance, not for actions or choices but rather for appreciative attitudes.[13] To be valuable is to be worthy of being valued in some way — that is, worthy of being the object of some appreciative response. This conception allows us to understand a kind of value that is not merely incommensurable but constitutively incomparable, because it is properly appreciated by a response that essentially involves a refusal to make comparisons, an insistence on cherishing its object in isolation from others.

Love is just such an attitude. We treasure the object of our love as special, not by comparing him favorably with alternative love objects, but rather by focusing appreciative attention solely on him, shunning any thought

---

12 Iris Murdoch, "The Sublime and the Good", in *Existentialists and Mystics: Writings on Philosophy and Literature*, ed. Peter Conradi (New York: Penguin, 1997), 205-220, p. 215.

13 I borrow this conception of value from Elizabeth Anderson, *Value in Ethics and Economics* (Cambridge, MA: Harvard University Press, 1993).

of alternatives. Each person is special in the sense that he deserves to be valued singularly in this manner, as he is in himself. In this sense, each person can be literally beyond compare.

I believe that deserving to be valued singularly, without comparison, is what Kant had in mind when he spoke of a person as a self-existent end. The appearance of paradox in this doctrine is due to a confusion between being valued singularly, without comparison, and being evaluated as singular in comparison with others. The latter cannot be deserved by everyone, obviously, but the former can.

Thus far I have said that love is a noncomparative response to another's personhood as vividly perceived through the medium of those characteristics which we are said to love the person for. But what can be said about the response itself? How do we respond to another person in loving him?

For an answer to this question, I draw on a comparison that many philosophers find counterintuitive — namely, a comparison between love and Kantian respect. The comparison shouldn't be counterintuitive, I claim, because love is a moral emotion: in particular, it is the emotion by which moral sensibilities are first implanted in children and by which the moral sensibilities of adults are enlivened or, if necessary, revived. If loving someone were not somehow akin to respecting him, love could not be the moral education that it is.[14]

Now, Kant characterizes the response to a person that he calls respect by saying that it "checks" or "arrests" our self-seeking motives, which might otherwise move us to use the person merely as a means to our ends.[15] I think that love resembles respect in being an arresting awareness of another's value — a description that I intend to be understood both phenomenologically and functionally. Like wonder, awe, and amazement, these emotions give us the feeling of being pulled up short, brought to attention, riveted, transfixed. And in each of these emotions some other, distracting motivational tendency is actually being arrested, though it is not the same tendency in every case. Whereas respect arrests our self-interested

---

14 Harry Frankfurt says, "The function of love … is not to make people good." I disagree. (Or I would insist that making people good is, if not the function of love, at least one of its effects.) Frankfurt's statement appears in "The Dear Self", *Philosophers' Imprint* 1, no. 1 (2001), http://www.philosophersimprint.org/001000/

15 Actually, Kant says that what respect "checks" is our self-love, but Kant isn't thinking of love at all, in my view. 'Self-love' for Kant means "self-interest".

designs on a person, love arrests our emotional defenses against him, leaving us emotionally vulnerable to him.[16] In colloquial terms, loving someone lays our heart open to him, leaving us emotionally disarmed and susceptible to all manner of other emotions toward him.

This difference between respect and love is reflected in their motivational potentials. Because respect for a person checks our self-interested motives toward him, its motivational force tends toward restraint, abstinence, and noninterference. Because love for a person checks our emotional defenses against him, its motivational force favors involvement and engagement. Respecting someone, we take care not to do various things to him or to let various things happen to him; loving someone, we are open to caring about him in all sorts of ways.

The foregoing descriptions of love are too abstract to convey the feeling, of course; indeed, their abstractness serves only to make them seem phenomenologically false. I have tried to describe the feeling of love by saying that it is an arresting awareness of value, similar to other arresting responses such as wonder and awe, and that it arrests our emotional defenses, so that it results in an opening of the heart. I hope that these admittedly vague and metaphorical descriptions find at least some resonance in the reader's experience of love. I have tried to think of a familiar experience that will similarly resonate with my claim that this arresting awareness of value is, more specifically, an awareness of personhood. Oddly enough, the best example I can find is one that doesn't involve actual personhood at all: it's the experience of loving a dog.

It's not so odd, really. Precisely because a dog isn't a person, we can more readily notice when we start to see him as one. If he's the right dog and we have the right rapport with him, we come to see him looking back at us with what seems like intelligent self-awareness, which makes his habitual obedience seem more like respect for us, and his instinctual affection more like love. Looking into his eyes, we seem to see *someone there*, someone who can reciprocate these interpersonal emotions. And having seen someone there, we are susceptible to feeling that form of love which I have described

---

16 I suspect that aesthetic appreciation is an arresting awareness in the same sense, responding to the beauty of an artwork, e.g., in a way that leaves us emotionally vulnerable to its content. I believe that Kant describes respect as an arresting awareness. What is arrested in respect, according to Kant, is self-love — though I believe that 'love' is a misnomer, since what Kant has in mind is self-interest.

as fiercer than mere benevolent affection. We are also susceptible to feeling not just irritated by the dog, if he misbehaves, but betrayed, because we have trusted him, when we should have known that all there is to trust is his training.

I am quite sure that my feelings for my late poodle were a response to the experience of seeing someone there in his eyes. In clearheaded moments, I don't believe that there really was someone there, but I am still under the illusion after his death, remembering him as I would a deceased person — not a lost toy for which I felt a fond attachment but a beloved personal presence, even though he was only a dog.

Murdoch's description of love as the realization that something is real other than oneself may seem to imply that loving oneself is either unavoidable or impossible.[17] If things other than oneself are the ones whose reality is difficult to realize, then perhaps one's own reality is obvious and the realization constitutive of love is unavoidable in reference to oneself. Or perhaps one can never have the requisite realization in reference to oneself, because it must be the realization of reality in something else. In fact, however, I think that Murdoch's description explains self-love more convincingly than the alternatives. Specifically, it better explains why loving oneself is possible but by no means easy, a moderately difficult accomplishment.

Of course, most people think well of themselves, and most also favor their own interests. If love were just a form of flattery or favoritism, then self-love would be virtually universal. But our test for whether people genuinely love themselves comes when we love them, thereby responding to their value in a way that models what self-love on their part would be. And when we love people, we frequently find that their self-flattery and self-favoritism fall somewhat short of love.

Genuine self-love is elusive because it requires a vivid awareness of one's personhood, consisting in one's rational autonomy. One can rarely avoid being vividly present to oneself as the conscious subject of feelings and behaviors, but one can easily be blinded to one's own autonomy or to the moral valence of that capacity. One can consequently raise emotional defenses against oneself, defenses that take the familiar forms of repression and dissociation. One feels threatened by one's unruly impulses, because one is blinded to one's own capacity to tame them with the force of respect

---

17 On the subject of self-love, see Frankfurt, "The Dear Self". I will have more to say about this essay in the Appendix, below.

and love, and so one is moved to deny having such impulses or being responsible for the behavior that might express them. Self-love enables one to accept the presence of unruly impulses, to accept oneself as subject to them, because it involves the vivid awareness of something in oneself that can be trusted to manage them. And self-love thereby facilitates the lifting of repression and the healing of dissociation.[18]

When I say that loving someone is a response to the value of rational autonomy, I am not saying that we love him for being rationally autonomous. My view, as I have said, is that the qualities "for" which we love someone are the qualities that serve as signs or symbols of his rational autonomy in our eyes. To my knowledge, this view is the only way to explain why we can love someone for his flaws.

Sometimes the recognition of a brushstroke as a flaw is what alerts us to its surroundings as a work of art, as having a value without which that stroke would be just another daub of paint. Similarly, an actor's portrayal of a character's weaknesses can be what makes the character seem real — really a person, that is, having those powers of rational autonomy against which human traits can stand out as weaknesses. A trait that would be merely a nuisance in another animal can be, in a person, the foil that casts his personhood into relief, the exception that proves the rule. We can love someone for his flaws, then, because our seeing them as flaws can be what alerts us to the fact that we are seeing a person, with the capacities against which they stand out as flaws.

My conception of love, when combined with the views of Darwall and Rosati, favors an Aristotelian conception of a person's interests. What it makes sense to care about out of love for a person is the unimpeded realization of his personhood, which might be described as his flourishing, in that sense of the term which is used to translate Aristotle's 'eudaimonia'. Caring about the self-realization of the beloved is not intrinsic to the emotion of love itself; it is one of the further responses to which love makes us susceptible by disarming our emotional defenses. But it is the further response that most naturally ensues when our defenses have been disarmed in response to the value of the beloved in himself, since it is a desire to see that value brought to its fullest realization.

---

18 It also facilitates self-forgiveness.

We can observe this aspect of love in the feelings of parents for their young adult children, who are just coming into the full realization of their personhood. What I found natural to care about out of love for my adolescent children was, to begin with, that they find direction — goals in pursuit of which to exercise their powers. Nothing makes parents of young adults fret more than seeing their children adrift.[19] And once my children adopted some directions — and there were many different directions over the years — I found myself caring about their progress in those directions, no matter how little intrinsic value I might have been inclined to see there in advance. In a quick succession of years, I became deeply interested in lacrosse and Morris dancing, poetry slams and photography, and specifically in the accomplishments of a particular midfielder, Morris dancer, poet, or photographer, because these were the directions that my children had set for themselves. Of course, I eventually learned to appreciate some of these accomplishments intrinsically: I would realize with amazement that I was cheering as my son walloped a schoolmate with a metal stick, or that I was applauding choreography that previously would have struck me as no more than quaint. But I learned to appreciate these accomplishments, to begin with, because they were the ones that my children had chosen to cultivate. In other words, I learned to appreciate them out of love for my children.

These examples introduce three distinct but related values. First is the value of my children as persons. Next is the value of their good, which consists in whatever it makes sense to care about out of an appreciation for their value. I have suggested that the relevant mode of appreciation is love, and that what it makes sense to care about out of love for them is the realization of their autonomy — their exercise of the capacity to which my love is an appreciative response. In loving my sons, I respond to the powers constitutive of their personhood, and it then makes sense for me to care about their exercise of those powers, bringing their personhood to fruition. And their exercise of those powers, because it is that which it makes sense to me to care about out of appreciation of their value, is what constitutes their good.

---

19 Frankfurt makes a similar point in "The Dear Self", p. 10. (I quote the relevant passage at n. 26, below.) See also Frankfurt's essay "On the Usefulness of Final Ends", in his *Necessity, Volition, and Love* (Cambridge: Cambridge University Press, 1999), pp. 82-94.

Finally, there is the value of the ends in whose pursuit my children realized their autonomy. Caring about their ends is not quite the same as caring about their interests, though the two are deeply entangled. Playing lacrosse wasn't essential to my son's good: he could have exercised his powers in many other pursuits instead. But of course his autonomy could be properly exercised only in pursuits of his own choosing, and lacrosse was what he chose. I might have thought that lacrosse was a bad choice — indeed, a choice inimical to his interests, if I had thought that it would expose him to serious injury that would damage his prospects for autonomous pursuits in the future. In that case, I would have seen a conflict of value between his interests and his ends. This conflict would have been of the maddening sort that arises between values that are at least partly traceable to a common source.

The value of my son's end, playing lacrosse, was distinct from the value of his good, which was the realization of his autonomy. But these two values were at least partly connected, because his end derived some of its value from its being that in pursuit of which he chose to realize his autonomy — a direction in which he decided that his flourishing would unfold. I will have more to say about this connection in a moment.

Because respect and love respond to the value of a person, they are responses out of which we do or want things for the person's sake, thereby taking the person as our end. But what we do or want for the person's sake out of love is rather different from what we do or want out of respect. The difference is perhaps clearest in our stance toward the person's ends.

Respect for a person restrains us from interfering with his pursuit of his ends, and it can also restrain us from taking a stance of indifference to whether he has the wherewithal to pursue them. But insofar as we merely respect someone, his success in attaining his ends doesn't matter to us, so long as we leave him free to do his best. I have now suggested that love engenders a different attitude, leading us to care about the full realization of personhood in the beloved through his autonomous endeavors. I have illustrated this suggestion by describing our tendency to care about the endeavors of someone we love even if we see no intrinsic value in them.

I think that this manifestation of love occurs in the reflexive case as well — that is, in love for oneself. Of course, one is already motivated toward one's ends simply by virtue of having adopted them, to begin with: they are things that one wants, or at least aims to attain. And yet there are plenty of things that one wants or aims to attain without feeling that they really matter or that attaining them is of any importance. One doesn't take them seriously or care about them deeply. But if one loves oneself, then one will care about one's ends, not merely out of having adopted them as ends, in the first place, but also out of concern for the realization of one's autonomy through the pursuit and attainment of whatever ends one has adopted. One will have, in other words, a second-order concern for one's ends, out of love for the self who has chosen to invest his autonomy in pursuing them. And this second-order concern will transform one's ends from objects that one merely desires or aims at into objects about which one genuinely cares.

(The idea of such a transformation by second-order attitudes will be familiar from the work of Harry Frankfurt. And I think that the point I have just made about self-love, in particular, is present in some of Frankfurt's writings, though not in the writings primarily devoted to the topic of love. In the Appendix to this chapter, I examine the relation between Frankfurt's views on the subject and my own.)

I now return, at last, to the argument against escapist suicide, which occasioned the foregoing reflections on love and personal good. Do these reflections provide materials for repairing the argument?

On the conception of personal good that I have developed, a person's good does not include his happiness essentially: it includes his happiness only because happiness is one of his ends. His good consists in the full realization of his rational autonomy, which is what would make sense to care about out of appreciation for his value as a person. His happiness makes sense to care about out of love for the person only because it is one of the ends in pursuit of which he must fully realize his autonomy. Indeed, it makes sense for *him* to care about, rather than merely desire, only out love for himself, and only as one of many ends whose pursuit would bring his autonomy to full realization.

Here escapist suicide impinges on the relevant concerns in the irrational manner that I described at the outset. In caring about our own autonomy out of self-love, we care about its full realization, which cannot come in the pursuit of a single end such as happiness, much less in the exercise of a single, one-time choice such as suicide. Out of respect for a person we can restrain ourselves from interfering with a single choice on his part, but in loving the person we want to see his autonomy brought to fruition more broadly. And because our own happiness is worth caring about only out of self-love, it is worth caring about only out of an appreciative response that extends to more than any one exercise of autonomy. Insofar as a person still has a variety of ends that he is capable of pursuing autonomously, they make sense for him to care about out of self-love. But of course suicide brings all of his pursuits to an end. Suicide therefore thwarts the concern out of which happiness is worth wanting in the way that entrenches it in the person's good. In sum, self-interested suicide is irrational.

My own view is that hastening death becomes morally appropriate only in the context of deterioration or suffering that compromises autonomy to an extent that can make talk of suicide inappropriate. But my conclusion about self-interested suicide can be stated more generally so as to encompass end-of-life decisions that are not solely on the shoulders of the prospective decedent. The conclusion is that we should not favor ending someone's life out of sympathy for him or concern for his happiness; we should favor ending his life only when we can do so out of love.

I think that sympathy or benevolence toward a loved one can tempt us to indulge his expressed wish for assistance in dying even when our love for him rebels at the thought. Such are the cases in which we should hesitate, in my view. We must of course distinguish carefully between loving perception of the person as he really is and attachment to him as he formerly was. Reluctance to let go of what is already gone should not determine our response. But neither should sympathy or benevolence, when they are not seconded by genuine, clear-sighted love.

I have elsewhere endorsed the slogan 'death with dignity', which I interpret as meaning "death while dignity is still mostly intact, before it suffers further, irrevocable deterioration".[20] Unfortunately, however, the word 'dignity' is not generally understood in the morally relevant, Kantian sense; it is often used to denote grounds of self-esteem, such as youth, good looks, and independence. Maybe, then, I should advocate retiring the slogan 'death with dignity' in favor of 'death with love', meaning "death only as love would allow".

---

20 See "A Right of Self-Termination?", chapter 3 of this volume.

Appendix: Harry Frankfurt on Caring

On the topic of "caring", Frankfurt says: [21]

> We often devote our time and effort and other resources to the pursuit of goals that we desire to attain because we are convinced of their intrinsic value but that we do not really consider to be of any importance to us. ... Suppose someone is planning to attend a concert that is to be devoted to music he particularly enjoys. There are easily imaginable circumstances in which he might emphatically and sincerely declare that, although he certainly does want to go to the concert, it is not something that he regards as being at all important to him. Consider the following scenario. The prospective concertgoer is asked by a close friend for an important favor. Doing the favor will make it impossible for him to get to the concert. He agrees gladly to do the favor, but incidentally mentions to his friend that doing it will require him to change his plans for the evening. Upon hearing this, his friend becomes confused and apologetic, expresses a reluctance to impose upon his good-natured readiness to forgo the concert, and begins to withdraw the request for the favor. At this point, the music lover interrupts him, saying: "Don't worry about the possibility that you may be taking too much advantage of my friendship for you. The fact is that going to this concert is not at all important to me. I really don't care about missing it."

In order for this person to care about going to the concert, according to Frankfurt, his desire to go would have to be such as to persist even if he decides not to, and "the persistence of his desire must be due to the fact that he is unwilling to give it up" — that is, "the fact that he is disposed to support and sustain his desire". [22] Caring thus has the hierarchical structure that is familiar from so much of Frankfurt's work in moral psychology.

Frankfurt says that caring about things matters to us independently of whether they are intrinsically worth caring about. It matters because it is the means by which we give our lives coherence and unity, by supporting and sustaining some of our desires over time: [23]

> Suppose we cared about nothing. In that case, we would be creatures with no active interest in establishing or sustaining any thematic continuity in our volitional lives. We would not be disposed to make any effort to maintain any of the interests, aims, and ambitions by which we are from time to time moved. ... From our point of view as agents ... whatever coherence

---

21 Harry G. Frankfurt, "On Caring", in *Necessity, Volition, and Love*, 155–180, p. 159.
22 Ibid., p. 160.
23 Ibid., p. 162.

or unity might happen to come about ... would be merely fortuitous and inadvertent. It would not be the result of any deliberate or guiding intent on our part. Desires and volitions of various hierarchical orders would come and go; and sometimes they might last for a while. But in the design and contrivance of their succession we ourselves would be playing no concerned or defining role.

Because caring about things is our way of giving coherence and unity to our lives, Frankfurt believes, it has an importance beyond that of the particular things that we care about: "The value to us of the fact that we care about various things does not derive simply from the value or the suitability of the objects about which we care. Caring is important to us for its own sake, insofar as it is the indispensably foundational activity through which we provide continuity and coherence to our volitional lives. Regardless of whether its objects are appropriate, our caring about things possesses for us an inherent value by virtue of its essential role in making us the distinctive kind of creatures that we are."[24]

The choice of objects to care about can thus be governed by the value of caring itself rather than the value of the objects:

> What makes it more suitable, then, for a person to make one object rather than another important to himself? It seems that it must be the fact that it is *possible* for him to care about the one and not about the other, or to care about the one in a way which is more important to him than the way in which it is possible for him to care about the other. ... The person does not care about the object because its worthiness commands that he do so. On the other hand, the worthiness of the activity of caring commands that he choose an object which he will be able to care about.[25]

Now, Frankfurt doesn't say exactly why it matters or should matter to us that our lives have continuity, coherence, and unity. But he does say that it will matter to us insofar as we love ourselves:[26]

> Parents express their love ... by doing what they can to ensure that their children actually have genuine interests and are therefore not condemned to lives that are chaotically fragmented and empty of meaning. Thus, their concern may extend also to helping their children to become capable of

---

24 Ibid., pp. 162-163.
25 Harry G. Frankfurt, "The Importance of What We Care About", in his *The Importance of What We Care About* (Cambridge: Cambridge University Press, 1988), p. 94.
26 Frankfurt, "The Dear Self", p. 10.

loving, to encouraging and assisting them to find love. This suggests that a person who loves nothing may nonetheless be able to show that he loves himself by attempting to alter whatever personal characteristics may impair his capacity to love and by making suitable efforts to find things to love.

Frankfurt conceives of love as a selfless identification with, and concern for, the interests of the beloved. In the essay from which this last quotation is drawn, he says that "the true interests of anyone … are defined and determined by what he loves."[27] Yet he goes on to say, in the quoted passage, that love for someone gives rise to a concern for something beyond what he loves — a concern, that is, for his having something *to* love, so that his life will have coherence and unity. And the value for the beloved of having something to love in the first place cannot be explained by his loving anything antecedently. Hence, Frankfurt seems to presuppose a "true interest" on the part of the beloved that is prior to that which is defined and determined by what he loves.

I would say that the interest in question is the interest that every person has in the fullest realization of his rational autonomy, which is in his interest because it is what would be most natural to want for his sake, out of love for him. A person most fully realizes himself as a person by having sustained and coherent pursuits, and so his caring about some pursuits in this fashion is what would make sense for anyone to want out of an appreciative response to his personhood. Like Frankfurt, I believe that it is what we want for our children, out of love for them; and I agree with Frankfurt that it is also what we want for ourselves, out of self-love.

---

27 Ibid., p. 8.

5. Family History[1]

When I received my maternal grandfather's birth certificate from the General Register Office in London, I found that the space for the mother's signature had been completed in the same official hand as the rest of the certificate. It read, "The mark of Golda, Mother" next to a tiny, tentative x. Golda's mark, similarly annotated, appears on the birth certificates of my grandfather's next older brother and younger sister, who were also born in London, each at a different address in the East End.

My great-grandparents had arrived in London, with two children, sometime before 1891, the date on the birth certificate of their first English-born child. Different versions of family lore trace them variously to Minsk, Kobryn, and Brest-Litovsk, although the best guess may be that they moved from one location in Ukraine to another before deciding to leave altogether. After the birth of their fifth child, they left London for New York, the father sailing in 1895, the mother and children a year later. On the ship's manifest, archived at Ellis Island, he is listed as Nathan Saltman, thirty-two years old, a cabinetmaker from Russia.

My grandfather attended the City University of New York and became a teacher in the New York City public schools. One of his daughters followed him into that profession; the other daughter, my mother, became a school librarian. I and my two brothers are university professors.

1   This is the accepted manuscript of an article originally published by Taylor and Francis in *Philosophical Papers* 34 (2005): 357-378, http://dx.doi.org/10.1080/05568640509485163 For comments and discussion, I am grateful to Jason Stanley, Connie Rosati, Thaddeus Metz, and Ward Jones. For information about donor conception, I am grateful to Diane Allen of InfertilityNetwork.org. Thanks also to Joanna Rose, Myfanwy Walker, Caroline Lorbach, Narelle Grech, Bill Cordray, Eric Blyth, and John Triseliotis.

I assume that my great-grandfather left Ukraine to escape conscription into the Czar's army, or some equally unpalatable fate devised for the Jews. I do not know why the family left England for the United States. Judging from the changes of address recorded on the children's birth certificates, I imagine that work in the Jewish furniture factories in the East End afforded only a precarious living. No doubt, the parents were looking for something better.

I and my brothers are the beneficiaries of that search: we have the "something better" that our great-grandparents were looking for. It has turned out to include the luxury of writing essays such as this for a living, three short generations after a time when births in the family were certified with an *x*.

That I am the great-grandson of Russian Jewish immigrants, that I enjoy the fruits of their strivings — this much I know with certainty. I also know that I inherited not just the fruits but the striving, too. What I don't know is how to understand that latter piece of my inheritance. Was it passed down entirely through my mother's upbringing by her father, and my upbringing by her? Or is the push in my personality a genetic endowment, from great-grandparents who twice pushed on?

A formal photograph of Nathan and Golda, dated 1918 and signed "Sincerely, Ma and Pa", hangs on the wall of our living room, next to a photo of my wife's paternal grandmother as a child, with her parents and siblings. My great-grandparents stand in their best clothes, looking awkwardly resolute; my wife's great-grandparents sit on a rustic front porch in Tennessee, looking more than a little like hillbillies. I think of these pictures as representing the eclectic ancestry of my children.

My children have inherited attitudes and lifeways from these ancestors, but they would have received such a cultural inheritance from anyone who had reared the people who reared them, or the people who had reared those people, and so on — anyone connected to them by the ancestral of the "parenting" relation, whether or not it corresponded to the relation of biological ancestry. Does it matter that their cultural inheritance came, in fact, from the same sources as their genes? If it had come from different sources, would their ancestry have mattered to them, divergent as it would then have been from their cultural past?

Naturally, my children's ancestry would still have mattered in that it would have influenced many of their characteristics, from their appearance to their aptitudes. What I'm asking, though, is whether their ancestry would or should have mattered in their eyes. Would they have had any reason to care about their progenitors — about knowing who their progenitors were or knowing them, as we philosophers say, by acquaintance?

Many adoptees think so. They go to heroic lengths to find their biological families, impelled by what they describe as a deep and unrelenting need.[2] But maybe they are just confused, because of living in a culture that is itself confused about the importance of biological ties. Maybe adoptees could be brought to see the insignificance of ancestry, if only they were sufficiently rational and realistic.

We had better hope so. For our society has embarked on a vast social experiment in producing children designed to have no human relations with some of their biological relatives. Conceived of anonymously donated sperm or eggs, these children are permanently severed from all or part of their biological past.[3]

---

2   A recent literature review concludes: "Following conservative estimates of more recent studies in countries with open records policies, about 50% of all adopted persons will, at some point in their life, search for their birth parents" (Ulrich Müller and Barbara Perry, "Adopted Persons' Search for and Contact with Their Birth Parents I: Who Searches and Why?", *Adoption Quarterly* 4 [2001]: 5-37, p. 8). These numbers have recently been increasing (p. 9), perhaps in response to greater awareness and acceptance of such searches.

   The offspring of donated sperm and eggs have also begun to search for their biological families, often via the Internet. See, for example, the Donor Sibling Registry (http://www.donorsiblingregistry.com); the Donor Offspring, Parent & Sibling Registry and Search Page (http://www.amfor.net/DonorOffspring); the "Donor Offspring" page of the Donor Conception Support Group of Australia (http://www.dcsg.org.au); and the UK Donor Link Voluntary Information Exchange and Contact Register (http://www.ukdonorlink.org.uk). See also David Plotz, *The Genius Factory: The Curious History of the Nobel Prize Sperm Bank* (New York: Random House, 2005). See also an op-ed entitled "Give Me My Own History", David Gollancz (*The Guardian*, May 19, 2002, http://www.theguardian.com/society/2002/may/20/comment.comment). On the similarities between donor conception and adoption, see Eric Blyth, Marilyn Crawshaw, Jean Haase, and Jennifer Speirs, "The Implications of Adoption for Donor Offspring Following Donor-Assisted Conception", *Child & Family Social Work* 6 (2001): 295-304.

3   In discussing gamete donation, I am going to gloss over the many variations in this practice, in which single adults, homosexual couples, or infertile heterosexual couples cause a child to be conceived with donated sperm, donated eggs, or both, often but not always with the help of in vitro fertilization or gestational surrogacy. Locutions designed to maintain strict neutrality among these variants would be unwieldy, and so I avoid them in favor of shorter but admittedly less precise locutions. For example, I generally speak of donor parents and custodial parents in the plural, although there may be only one of each. Generating the relevant disjunction of variants is left as an exercise for the reader.

   Cases of gamete donation often have other potentially controversial aspects. For example, there is often only one custodial parent, or no custodial parent of one sex or the other. Creating children with the intention that they not have a custodial father, or alternatively a custodial mother, is potentially just as problematic as creating children divorced from their biological origins. But these problems are a topic for another paper.

The experiment of creating these children is supported by a new ideology of the family, developed for people who want to have children but lack the biological means to "have" them in the usual sense. The new ideology has to do with the sense in which the resulting children will have families. It says that these children will have families in the only sense that matters, or at least in a sense that is good enough.

Clearly, it has turned out to be less than enough for any adopted person who goes in search of a biological family. The new ideology of the family is rarely mentioned in this context. The ideology isn't mentioned, I imagine, because it isn't needed to justify traditional adoption, in which people volunteer to replace biological parents who are unavailable, unwilling, or unfit to care for a child they have already conceived. The child needs to be parented by someone, and it cannot or should not be parented by its biological parents, for reasons that would outweigh any value inhering in biological ties. An ideology belittling the value of such ties is not needed to justify entrusting this child to adoptive parents.

The new ideology of the family is needed rather for cases in which people wanting to parent a child cause one to be conceived with donated gametes. That this child cannot be parented by one or both of its biological parents is not a disadvantage that its custodial parents volunteer to mitigate; it was a desideratum that guided them in creating the child, to begin with. Not being attached to a partner with whom they could be fertile, they needed a child who was correlatively unattached, a child already disowned by at least one of its biological parents. Rather than adopt a child whose ties to its biological parents had been ruptured after conception, they intentionally created one for whom those ties were ruptured antecedently. This choice would be morally problematic if biological ties were genuinely meaningful. Hence the need for an ideology that denies their meaning.

These remarks are admittedly polemical, and they will no doubt offend some readers. Whether there is anything to them depends on whether there is significant value in being parented by one's biological parents or, more generally, having human relations with one's biological relatives. The idea of such a value can hardly be considered unusual, given that it is enshrined in the United Nations Convention on the Rights of the Child. Article 7, paragraph l, states: "The child shall be registered immediately after birth and shall have the right from birth to a name, the right to acquire a nationality and, as far as possible, the right to know and be cared for by his or her parents."[4] The rights enunciated in this provision strike me as important, and this essay takes a few tentative steps toward explaining why.

I take only a few steps because I want to skirt many of the considerations that catch the eye on a first glance at the topic. The topic of our biological origins is littered with mythical or symbolic thoughts, about blood and bone and seed and such. I want to pick my way around these thoughts, in search of some realistic and rational considerations. My reason for being so cautious is that doubts about reproductive technology are often written off to fear and superstition. I want to avoid raising any considerations that might be dismissed on those grounds.

My caution in this regard will lead me to overlook many considerations that I see as genuinely meaningful. What is most troubling about gamete donation is that it purposely severs a connection of the sort that normally informs a person's sense of identity, which is composed of elements that must bear emotional meaning, as only symbols and stories can. To downplay the symbolic and mythical significance of severing a child's connections to its biological parents is therefore to misrepresent what is

---

4   The Convention is posted at http://www.ohchr.org/en/professionalinterest/pages/crc.aspx See Eric Blyth and Abigail Farrand, "Anonymity in Donor-Assisted Conception and the UN Convention on the Rights of the Child", *International Journal of Children's Rights* 12 (2004): 89-104. The *Implementation Handbook for the Convention on the Rights of the Child* makes clear that the term "parents" in this clause includes biological parents in the first instance, and that the Convention therefore militates against the practice of anonymous gamete donation (Rachel Hodgkin and Peter Newell, *Implementation Handbook for the Convention on the Rights of the Child* [UNICEF, revised edition 2002], pp. 117-119).

For some social-scientific and legal perspectives, with further references, see Michael Freeman, "The New Birth Right? Identity and the Child of the Reproduction Revolution", *The International Journal of Children's Rights* 4 (1996): 273-297; A. J. Turner and A. Coyle, "What Does It Mean to Be a Donor Offspring? The Identity Experiences of Adults Conceived by Donor Insemination and the Implications for Counselling and Therapy", *Human Reproduction* 15 (2000): 2041-2051; Lucy Frith, "Gamete Donation and Anonymity: The Ethical and Legal Debate", *Human Reproduction* 16 (2001): 818-824; *Truth and the Child: A Contribution to the Debate on the Warnock Report*, ed. Nigel Bruce, Ann K. Mitchell, and Kate Priestley (Edinburgh: Family Care, 1988); *Truth and the Child 10 Years On: Information Exchange in Donor Assisted Conception*, ed. Eric Blyth, Marilyn Crawshaw, and Jennifer Speirs (Birmingham: British Association of Social Workers, 1998).

The material cited here argues that donor-conceived offspring should have access to information about their biological parents. In this paper I argue for a stronger conclusion — that donor conception is wrong. In my view, the reasons for concluding that children should have access to information about their biological parents support the stronger conclusion that, other things being equal, children should be raised by their biological parents. For many children already born, other things are not at all equal, and adoption is therefore desirable; but as I argue below, other things are indeed equal for children who have not yet been conceived.

really going on, if not because the symbols and stories are literally true then at least because they are truly part of the human psyche.

But to speak of the human psyche in such terms is already to verge on superstition in the eyes of those who consider themselves enlightened. Although I will briefly reintroduce some of these terms at the end of my essay, I will first try to address the enlightened in their own rationalistic terms.

An argument against the use of donated gametes risks giving offense because it seems to raise doubts about particular children as to whether they should have been born. But talk about whether someone should or should not have been born is confused and confusing.[5]

'Should' and 'ought' express norms that tell us what to do. In addition to these norms recommending or requiring action, there are values attaching to objects and events, warranting various modes of appreciation for them. Events can be felicitous, deplorable, or regrettable, for example; persons, places, or things can be beautiful or ugly, admirable or contemptible, lovable or hateful, and so on. If you expect the world to deliver perfectly congruent norms and values — that is, if you expect that insofar as something is beautiful or admirable or lovable, its coming into existence will be a felicitous event, or its creation will be a right action — then you are bound to be disappointed. There are beautiful things whose creation is a grievous wrong (mushroom clouds), disgusting things whose coming into existence is fortunate (feces), regrettable events that are right to bring about (the death of an attacker), and so on.

Matters are further complicated by the possibility of conflict between values that attach to types and values that attach to individual tokens of them. My wedding ring may be precious to me even though it is of an inferior type, neither beautiful nor well-wrought nor of any significant monetary value; irises are gorgeous although one is just as good as another. If you expect the world to serve up only precious individuals of precious types, and vice versa, then you are bound to be disappointed once again.

To say that someone should or should not have been born mixes normative categories in a way that sows confusion about the object of

---

5   The arguments of this section are superseded by "Persons in Prospect", chapter 6 of this volume, especially part III, "Love and Nonexistence". I now regard the present arguments as inadequate.

assessment. Does this statement assess the person, the event of his coming into existence, or the act of creating him? And does it make an assessment with respect to him individually or with respect to some type that he instantiates?

Suppose we judge that people should not have more children than they can adequately care for. Have we implied that there are children who should not have been born? Yes, of course, if that statement means just that some children are born after their parents should have stopped having children. Yes, too, if it means that the birth of a child destined to be neglected is a regrettable kind of event. But we have not implied, of any particular child, that his existence should be regretted or that his birthday should not be celebrated. Loving an individual child and rejoicing in his existence is perfectly consistent with thinking it wrong for parents like his to have had so many children. And if you expect the world to spare you from this sort of evaluative complexity, then you are in for the biggest disappointment of all.

Much as we love disadvantaged children, we rightly believe that people should not deliberately create children who they already know will be disadvantaged. In my view, people who create children by donor conception already know — or already should know — that their children will be disadvantaged by the lack of a basic good on which most people rely in their pursuit of self-knowledge and identity formation. In coming to know and define themselves, most people rely on their acquaintance with people who are like them by virtue of being their biological relatives.

Philosophers should not have to be reminded that living things tend to resemble their biological relatives. After all, the philosophical term for indefinable similarities is 'family resemblance'. Though much has been written by philosophers about family resemblance in this technical sense, little has been written about literal resemblance within families, which is, after all, the paradigm case of technical family resemblance.

The philosophical concept of family resemblance is that of a similarity that can be immediately recognized but not readily analyzed or defined. Many of our concepts have their extension determined by family resemblance among their instances. To have such a family resemblance concept is just to have the ability to know an instance when we see one, without being able to say how we know it.

Although there is only one of me, I have a self-concept of the family-resemblance kind. This self-concept is not the singular concept by which I pick out the one and only me; it's my concept for the personal type of which I happen to be the only instance but to which a doppelgänger would belong, if I had one. I would recognize a doppelgänger under this concept, by our family resemblance.

Much of what I know about myself is contained in this family-resemblance concept and cannot be articulated. I know that I am *like this*, where the import of 'this' is encoded in the self-concept of which anyone just like me would be an instance. Hence much of my self-knowledge is, so to speak, knowledge about my family resemblance to myself. This family-resemblance knowledge about myself includes information not only about how I look but also about my personal manner, my styles of thinking and feeling, my temperament, and so on. This ellipsis is difficult to fill in without resort to figurative expressions, because family-resemblance information is unanalyzable by definition.

My concept of my self-resemblance contains much of my psychological knowledge about myself. Philosophers like to characterize folk psychology as a theory; in reality, however, most of folk psychology is an intuitive matter of knowing how to anticipate and deal with people *like that* — knowledge that is heavily dependent on family-resemblance concepts of personality types and behavioral styles. So it is with my folk-psychological self-understanding.

Finally, my family-resemblance concept of myself contains much of the self-knowledge by which I am guided in my efforts to cultivate and shape myself. I can articulate a few self-descriptions that indicate some directions of self-cultivation and contra-indicate others. I'm physically coordinated and I have a good sense of rhythm, so studying dance makes sense for me; I have a lousy memory and weak powers of mental computation, so studying chess is a bad idea. But many of my aspirations are directed at fulfilling family-resemblance concepts: they are aspirations to be *like that*, where 'that' denotes a type for which I have some paradigms or images but no explicit definition. And these aspirations are conditioned and channeled by family-resemblance knowledge as to how someone *like this* might or might not become *like that*.

I think that forming a useful family-resemblance concept of myself would be very difficult were I not acquainted with people to whom I bear a literal family resemblance. Knowing what I am like would be that much harder if

I didn't know other people like me. And if people bear me a literal family resemblance, then the respects in which they are like me will be especially important to my knowledge of what I am like, since they resemble me in respects that are deeply ingrained and resistant to change.

The difficulty of knowing what I am like is the topic of some suggestive remarks by Bernard Berenson in his *Sketch for a Self-Portrait*:[6]

> This self, what is it? For about seventy years I have been asking that question. Can one frame an idea of one's own personality, map it out, make a picture of it that is in any measure convincing to an inquiring and fairly honest mind? In my case it has not been possible. I know what people think of me, favourably and unfavourably, and I have a sense of what composite image of me ends by taking shape in the minds of acquaintances. In my own mind and heart there is little correspondence with this image, although I have learned to accept it as that in me, of me, to which others approach as to a treaty-port in old China or Japan. To myself I am an energy of a given force of radiation, and of a certain power of resistance; and I seem to be the same in these respects that I remember being when I completed my sixth year.
>
> … I wish I could have some image, a coherent image of my personality with a definite shape and clear outlines. It is hard enough to know how one looks, impossible to know what one is. We are left to infer it from what people say about us and what we accept, reject, repel and controvert in what we hear about ourselves. We cannot even get a notion remotely parallel to what we acquire by staring into a mirror. That is little enough, for we gaze fixedly, we pose, we search and ask 'is that me?' or 'is it that or that?'; and when it happens once in a blue moon that we look into a mirror unexpectedly we seldom recognize the image there appearing as a reflection of ourselves. Yet how definite is this corporeal shape compared with any sense of one's entire personality, so uncharted, of such wavering outlines, of such uncertain heights and depths!
>
> I have at times wondered what my instinctive and instantaneous reaction would be if I could meet myself for the first time. This has all but happened. More than once it occurred that somewhat absentmindedly I was mounting a broad staircase which at the landing had a pier-glass rising from floor to ceiling. I seemed to see coming toward me a figure not particularly to my taste, not at all corresponding to the type I instinctively liked; and this figure had an abstracted effaced expression that I should rather sidle away from than be drawn to. All this before recognizing that it was myself.

---

6   Bernard Berenson, *Sketch for a Self Portrait* (London: Robin Clark, 1991). The following quotations can be found at pp. 23, 27, and 67-68.

I find Berenson's remarks suggestive on several points. First, Berenson conceives of his personality as having a "shape" or "outline", like that of his physiognomy or physique. He thus suggests that his personality is an object not of analysis or description but rather of perceptual recognition, as if by family resemblance. Second, his psychological profile is inaccessible to introspection and therefore visible only from a detached perspective, as seen through other people's eyes. Finally, the usual technique for viewing himself externally, by looking in the mirror, proves inadequate because his reflection usually shows him in the act of self-presentation, striking a pose that is unlike his spontaneous self.

Presumably, the same difficulties arise for external self-inspection of his personality, for which mirrors are harder to come by and poses harder to see through.

If I want to see myself as another, however, I don't have to imagine myself as seen through other people's eyes: I just have to look at my father, my mother, and my brothers, who show me by way of family resemblance what I am like. For information about my appearance, they may not be as good a source as an ordinary mirror; but for information about what I am like as a person, they are the closest thing to a mirror that I can find.

If I want to know what a person *like this* can make of himself, I can look first at what my parents and grandparents made of themselves, or at the self-cultivation under way on the part of my brothers and cousins. The point is not that I necessarily can or should strive to be whatever my biological relatives have become, but rather that my own experiments-in-living (as Mill called them) are most informatively supplemented by experiments on the part of people who are relevantly like me. Our extended family is, as it were, a laboratory for carrying out experiments-in-living relevant to the lives of people like us.

When adoptees go in search of their biological parents and siblings, there is a literal sense in which they are searching for themselves. They are searching for the closest thing to a mirror in which to catch an external and candid view of what they are like in more than mere appearance. Not knowing any biological relatives must be like wandering in a world without reflective surfaces, permanently self-blind.

Children denied a knowledge of only one biological parent are not entirely cut off from this view of themselves, but they are cut off from one half of it. Their estrangement even from one parent, or from half-brothers and -sisters, must still be a deprivation, because it estranges them from people who would be familiar without any prior acquaintance, people with whom they would enjoy that natural familiarity which would be so revealing about themselves.

How odd it must be to go through life never knowing whether a sense of having met a man before is due to his being one's father. How tantalizing to know that there is someone who could instantly show one a living rendition of deeply ingrained aspects of oneself. How frustrating to know that one will never meet him!

When people deny the importance of biological ties, I wonder how they can read world literature with any comprehension. How do they make any sense of Telemachus, who goes in search of a father he cannot remember? What do they think is the dramatic engine of the Oedipus story? When the adoptive grandson of Pharaoh says, "I have been a stranger in a strange land", do they take him to be speaking merely as an Egyptian in the land of Midian?[7] How can they even understand the colloquy between Darth Vader and Luke Skywalker? Surely, the revelation "I am your father" should strike them as a bit of dramatic stupidity — a remark to be answered with "So what?"

Of course, these stories embody the mythical and symbolic values that I have promised not to invoke; but they also, and independently, illustrate a bit of common sense about the self-knowledge drawn from acquaintance with biological relatives. Telemachus, Oedipus, Moses, and even Luke Skywalker illustrate the centrality of this knowledge to the task of identity formation, and the centrality of that task to a meaningful human life. Through the ages, people unacquainted with their origins have been regarded as ill-equipped for a fundamental life-task and hence as dramatically, even tragically, disadvantaged.

As the offspring of donated gametes reach adulthood, they are rediscovering and reiterating the age-old wisdom about the importance of biological ties. In footnote 2, above, I have cited several online registries through which thousands of donor-conceived adults are seeking to contact their biological relatives. Britain has recently outlawed anonymous gamete donation, on the grounds of a child's right to know his or her parentage.

---

7   Exodus 2:22. The speaker is Moses, who not only *is* a stranger among the Midianites, where he has fled from Pharaoh's court, but *has been* a stranger all of his life, ever since his mother set him afloat on the Nile.

Donor offspring are beginning to protest their status as strangers in a strange land.

Acquaintance with a child's biological family can be a source of knowledge for people other than the child itself. The use of anonymously donated gametes can leave not just the child but also its custodial parents in the dark, and in ways that adversely affect their parenting.

Information relevant to self-cultivation is also relevant to the rearing of children. And that information is even more consequential for childrearing, because the growth of children is so dramatic in comparison with what is still possible once the age of self-cultivation has been attained. So much of what perplexes parents has to do with the nature whose unfolding they are trying to foster. How far can the child hope to reach and in which directions? What is the child unable to help being and what can it be helped to become? What will smooth its rough edges and what will just rub against the grain?

I would not want to have raised my son without having known my maternal grandfather, with whom he has so much in common. I would never have understood my daughter if I hadn't known her uncles, on both sides. And raising my children without knowing their mother — that would have been like raising them with one eye closed. It's not just my sympathetic knowledge of her that has helped me to understand them but also my understanding of her and me in relation to one another, since each child is a blend of qualities that were first blended in our relationship.

Some truths are so homely as to embarrass the philosopher who ventures to speak them. First comes love, then comes marriage, and then the proverbial baby carriage. Well, it's not such a ridiculous way of doing things, is it? The baby in that carriage has an inborn nature that joins together the natures of two adults. If those two adults are joined by love into a stable relationship — call it marriage — then they will be naturally prepared to care for the child with sympathetic understanding, and to show it how to recognize and reconcile some of the qualities within itself. A child naturally comes to feel at home with itself and at home in the world by growing up in its own family.

Human families are disrupted in various ways, by death or divorce or poverty or social upheavals. In these circumstances a child is entitled to be raised by parental figures who love it and love one another, even if they are not its biological parents. The child is also entitled to feel that it is the social equal of other children and that its parents are the equals of other parents. Here again, however, different evaluations are easily conflated or confused. To acknowledge that adopted children have missed something of human importance is not to disparage the children, their parents, or the love and mutual care among them. Similarly, we should not have to disparage anyone in order to acknowledge that the offspring of donated gametes will miss something important as well. And then the contrast between these cases — between compensating children for something they have already lost and creating children with the intention that they never have it — should lead us to question the morality of anonymous genetic donation.

The reason for resorting to donated gametes in many cases, of course, is the desire of an adult to have a biologically related child despite lacking a partner with whom he or she can conceive. And my arguments imply that having a biologically related child is of genuine value, as a potential source of self-knowledge for the parent. Yet whereas the parent will be just as fully related to the child as any mother or father, the child will know only half of its biological parentage. Surely, we don't believe that parents are entitled to make themselves slightly better off in some fundamental dimension by impoverishing their children in the same dimension. Why, then, should they be entitled to enlarge their own circle of consanguinity by creating children whose circle will be broken in half?

The answer to this question cannot be that the children will be compensated by receiving the gift of life. The so-called gift of life cannot compensate a child for congenital disadvantages, because it doesn't make the child better off than it would have been without them.[8]

Look at it this way. We cannot justify severing the child's ties to one of its parents by pointing out that, in order to avoid doing so, we would have had to omit creating the child altogether. This justification would portray separation from a biological parent as the lesser of two evils for the child, preferable to the greater evil of never having existed. But never having existed would not have been an evil for the child, because a nonexistent person suffers no evils.

To be sure, the child of a genetic donor is usually glad to have been born. But the fact that a child would be glad to have been born cannot justify us

---

8 I call it a "so-called gift" because it has no intended recipient. It is a "gift" that is launched into the void, where some as-yet-nonexistent person may snag it. Such untargeted benefits do not fit our usual concept of gift-giving. See also chapter 6, part II of this volume.

in conceiving it.[9] Congenitally handicapped people live rich and fulfilling lives into which they are glad to have been born, but a woman who is taking a teratogenic medication has an obligation not to conceive a child until she has stopped taking it. Waiting to conceive until she has stopped taking the medication will of course entail that the handicapped child she might have conceived will in fact never exist. Had she conceived that child, it might even have been thankful that she chose not to wait before conceiving. But the wrongness of deliberately conceiving a handicapped child cannot be mitigated by that child's future thankfulness. To offer such a justification would be to confuse two distinct questions.

One question asks, about a particular individual, whether the disadvantages of his life are so great as to outweigh the value for him of living. This is the question that someone answers by being glad to have been born or, alternatively, wishing that he hadn't been; but it is not the question that we face at the point of deciding whether to conceive a child. At that point there is no particular individual with respect to whom we can ask whether he would welcome or regret the kind of life we have to offer. So we have to compare there being a person who lives that kind of life, on the one hand, with there being so such person, on the other — abstractly quantified alternatives concerning no particular individual. Such a person, if he existed, would compare *his* living such a life with *his* never having lived — alternatives concerning him in particular. How he would choose between a disadvantaged life and nonexistence, as alternatives concerning him in particular, cannot dictate how we should choose between there being a person who faces such alternatives and there being none. Preferring a disadvantaged life as the only alternative to nonexistence may be a rational choice for him to make, and yet those alternatives may be such as no person should have to face. Indeed, the reason why there should be no person who has to face these alternatives is precisely that, once brought into existence facing them, he will find that his own individual nonexistence is the only alternative to his disadvantages.

Frankly, to criticize proponents of gamete donation for overselling the "gift of life" is to credit them with greater moral sensitivity than they generally show. Gamete donation is presented as affecting primarily the parents, by enabling them to "create families".

---

9   Here I am introducing the "non-identity problem" first discussed by Derek Parfit in *Reasons and Persons* (Oxford: Oxford University Press, 1984). I discuss this problem in parts II and III of chapter 6.

But the party of the first part in these transactions is surely the child. For the parent, the birth is the beginning of a particular life-stage; for the child it's the beginning of life itself — the beginning of a life that will extend far beyond the parents' control or ken. The question "Is this a good way to get a child?" cannot dominate the question "Is this a good way for a child to have been gotten?" And the latter question cannot be finessed on the grounds that a particular child could not have been gotten any other way, since the alternative for that child would have been a benign nonexistence.

Nor can the former question be given precedence on the grounds that gamete donation is the only way for the prospective parents to get a child. The alternative of adopting an already existing child is often available, and I have argued that it is morally preferable, because it provides a custodial family for a child already and independently destined to be alienated from its biological family. As I have mentioned, creating a new child designed to suffer that alienation is often preferred to adoption precisely because of the parents' interest in biological ties — an interest that they choose to further slightly in their own case by creating a person for whom the same interest will be profoundly frustrated. I regard this choice as morally incoherent.

What's more, there is the question of what moral weight attaches to a person's desire to procreate. Traditionally, that desire has been thought to ground a moral right to procreate only for those who are in a position to provide the resulting child with a family. According to the new ideology of the family, of course, virtually any adult is in a position to satisfy this requirement, since a family is whatever we choose to call by that name. But this new ideology is precisely what I am questioning. To defend the ideology on the grounds of a person's right to procreate would be question-begging. The right to procreate is conditional on the ability to provide the resulting child with a family; what counts as providing the child with a family in the relevant sense is a question that must be settled prior to any claim of procreative rights.[10]

---

10 Framing the considerations in this way makes clear their application to the case of single women who use artificial insemination to create children whom they intend to raise on their own. Children can of course be successfully reared by single mothers, if necessary. But children can be successfully reared, if necessary, in orphanages as well — a fact that cannot justify deliberately creating children with the intention of abandoning them to an orphanage. (Imagine a woman who would like to have the experience of conception and childbirth without incurring the responsibility for raising a child.) Just as the serviceability of orphanages cannot justify procreation in reliance on their services, so the serviceability of single parenting cannot justify the creation of children with the intention that they grow up without fathers of any kind.

I am inclined to think that a knowledge of one's origins is especially important to identity formation because it is important to the telling of one's life story, which necessarily encodes one's appreciation of meaning in the events of one's life.[11] I opened with the story of my Russian ancestors, whose search for something better I imagined to have culminated in my writing this essay. My family background includes many such stories, whose denouement I can see myself as undergoing or enacting. But do such family sagas have to be sagas of biological families? Let me approach this question by saying first what I think that stories do.[12]

Organizing events into the form of a story provides an understanding of them distinct from what would be provided by causal explanations. A well-constructed story recounts events in such a way as to lead us through a natural sequence of emotions, which is ultimately resolved in an emotional cadence that leaves us knowing how we feel about the events. We know how we feel because we have been through a sequence of feelings that is familiar to our emotional sensibilities; because we have arrived at a conclusory feeling, a state of emotional rest; and because our conclusory feeling takes all of the preceding events into its view.

To understand events in this emotional sense is to grasp their meaning — that is, what they mean to us in emotional terms. My finishing an essay on family histories is a meaningless event in a string of meaningless events unless and until I can embed it in a story that makes it an occasion for feeling ambitions achieved, fears allayed, sufferings redeemed — or pretensions punctured, for that matter. Of course, my own life provides narrative context for many of the events within it; but my family history provides an even broader context, in which large stretches of my life can take on meaning, as the trajectory of my entire education and career takes on meaning in relation to the story of my ancestors.

Adoptees can certainly find meaningful roles for themselves in stories about their adoptive families. Even so, they seem to have the sense of not knowing important stories about themselves, and of therefore missing some meaning implicit in their lives, unless and until they know their biological origins.

---

11 The importance of narrative self-knowledge is stressed by David Gollancz in the essay cited in note 2, above.

12 See my "Narrative Explanation", *The Philosophical Review* 112 (2003): 1-25.

Here the temptation of symbolic and mythical thinking grows, and I still want to avoid succumbing to it. Insofar as there is a realistic basis for valuing biological-family history, I suspect that it is the same as the basis I have already identified for self-knowledge — namely, the resemblances that hold within biological families. What rests on this basis is different, however, in the case of historical narrative.

Whereas direct acquaintance with biological relatives helps me to know what I am like, knowledge of family history helps me to understand what it means to be like this. The quality that sometimes makes me a malcontent seems to have impelled Nathan and Golda into the role of emigrants. The quality that makes me a homebody seems to have drawn their every migration toward a better urban homestead for their growing family. These different descriptions of our shared qualities endow those qualities with different meanings, by assigning them to the protagonists of different scenarios — the emigrants versus the malcontent, the homesteaders versus the homebody. The scenarios typical of these protagonists work their way toward different emotional resolutions, with corresponding differences in meaning.

I know that I have it in me to be a malcontent homebody, a grumbling stick-in-the-mud. Do I also have it in me to spurn one home for the prospect of a better one? Nathan and Golda did, according to their story, and it's because they did that am I here to ask the question, bearing their genetic legacy. Maybe, then, I should borrow a page from their book. The point, in any case, is that I could never have considered borrowing a page from that book if it had been permanently closed to me at birth.

How do I know that I have inherited these qualities from Nathan and Golda? I don't: it's all imaginative speculation. But such speculations are how we define and redefine ourselves, weighing different possible meanings for our characters by playing them out in different imagined stories. In these speculations, family history gives us inexhaustible food for thought. Why would we create children whose provision of possible self-understandings was poorer than our own?

I know that many people have no interest in their ancestry, no sense of kinship with their kin. These people define themselves in terms other than those which are descriptive of their relatives, and they pursue life stories disjoint from their family's history. But even these people benefit by knowing where they come from.

I think that someone who denies having anything in common with his biological relatives is either speaking figuratively or in denial. Almost all of us look and sound and feel and move like the people from whom we came: a genuine sport of nature is very rare. What is more likely is that a person's similarities to his relatives lie in aspects of himself that don't matter to him or that he dislikes and rejects. Not valuing commonalities is indeed a way of not having anything in common, figuratively speaking; it just isn't a way of literally having nothing in common.

Someone who doesn't value what he has in common with his relatives may think that he need never have known them in order to identify and cultivate those aspects of himself which he does value. But I doubt it. This person is likely to have defined himself as different from his relatives precisely because they served as ill omens of his possible futures, or at least as foils against which his contrasting qualities could attract his eye. Learning not to be like his relatives has still involved learning from them: if he had never known them, he might well have ended up more like them.

The point is that biological origins needn't be worth embracing in order to be worth knowing. Someone who doesn't know his relatives cannot even turn up his nose at them. The question for him is not "Shall I follow my forebears?" but "*Am* I following them?", and to this latter question he can never know the answer. He can have neither the satisfaction of continuing in their footsteps nor that of striking out on his own, because their footsteps have been effaced. To tell him that those obliterated footsteps weren't important for him is to tell what the experience of all times and cultures condemns as a lie.[13]

---

13 While this essay was in press, I learned of the following additional resource on donor conception: Since August 2005, New Zealand has required all donor-conceived births to be recorded in a Human Assisted Reproductive Technology (HART) Register (http:// www.dia.govt.nz/diawebsite.nsf/wpg_URL/Services-Births-Deaths-and-Marriages-Human-Assisted-Reproductive-Technology-%28HART%29-Register?OpenDocument). The HART Act requires that information about donors be made available to their offspring at age eighteen. In addition to the publications listed in note 3, see Jacqueline A. Laing and David S. Oderberg, "Artificial Reproduction, the 'Welfare Principle', and the Common Good", *Medical Law Review* 13 (2005): 328-356; and Alexina McWhinnie, "Gamete Donation and Anonymity: Should Offspring from Donated Gametes Continue to Be Denied Knowledge of Their Origins and Antecedents?", *Human Reproduction* 16 (2001): 807-817. Thanks to Rupert Rushbrooke for these references.

6. Persons in Prospect[1]

I. The Identity Problem

Derek Parfit calls it the *non*-identity problem.[2] It's the problem of how to treat future persons given that any attempt to treat them better may result instead in their never being born. For example, the people who will have inadequate resources in the twenty-second century because of our wastefulness today will owe their existence to human couplings that never would have occurred if we had lowered our thermostats and showered less often. As those future people commute on foot or read by candlelight, they will have to acknowledge that we couldn't have conserved resources for them, since our conserving would have prevented them from existing. Because the people affected by our wastefulness will not be identical to those who would have been affected by our conservation, there appear to be no future individuals for us to harm or benefit, whatever we do.

This description of the problem depends on an empirical assumption about the effects of our environmental policies on the makeup of the

---

1   This series was first published in *Philosophy & Public Affairs* 36 (2008): 221-288. It was written in conjunction with an undergraduate course on "Future Persons" taught at New York University in the fall of 2007. Thanks to the participants in the course and to Imogen Dickie, Jeff Sebo, and the editors of *Philosophy & Public Affairs.* Part I replaces the corresponding part in the published version.
2   Parfit first discussed the problem in "On Doing the Best for Our Children", in *Ethics and Population*, ed. Michael D. Bayles (Cambridge, MA: Schenkman, 1976), pp. 100-115. See also Robert Merrihew Adams, "Existence, Self-Interest, and the Problem of Evil", *Noûs* 13 (1979): 53-65; Gregory S. Kavka, "The Paradox of Future Individuals", *Philosophy & Public Affairs* 11 (1982): 93-112 ; and Thomas Schwartz, "Obligations to Posterity", in *Obligations to Future Generations*, ed. R. I. Sikora and Brian Barry (Philadelphia: Temple University Press, 1978), pp. 3-13. I will deal primarily with Parfit's discussion of the problem in Part IV of *Reasons and Persons* (Oxford: Oxford University Press, 1984).

population. I will argue that even if this empirical assumption were false, the problem would remain. Even if we could ensure that the people affected by our conserving resources were identical to the people affected by our wasting them, neither group could be harmed or benefited by what we do. I call it the *identity* problem, to indicate that it is a variant of Parfit's.

The Metaphysics of Survival

The identity problem, unlike the non-identity problem, hangs on controversial assumptions about the sameness of persons. It is fairly uncontroversial that two different pairs of gametes would result in the birth of two different persons, but it is more controversial whether one and the same pair of gametes would result in the birth of the same person irrespective of whatever else happened, which is the presupposition on which the identity problem is based. Moreover, Parfit himself believes that, even if the same person would be born from the same pair of gametes under different circumstances, that person would evolve, under different circumstances, so as to yield adults who weren't related in the ways that make sameness matter.

How sameness-of-person matters, Parfit addresses in the context of sameness across time, which constitutes a person's survival. When it comes to survival, according to Parfit, what matters — or, as he puts it, what is "worth caring about" — is the future existence of someone to whom we bear a relation of psychological connectedness and continuity. Parfit's definition of psychological connectedness begins with Locke's memory theory of personal identity: "Let us say", Parfit says, "that between X today and Y twenty years ago, there are *direct memory connections* if X can now remember having some of the experiences that Y had twenty years ago."[3] Parfit then expands on Locke's theory like this:

> We should ... revise [Locke's] view [of personal identity] so that it appeals to other facts. Besides direct memories, there are several other kinds of direct psychological connection. One such connection is that which holds between an intention and the later act in which this intention is carried out. Other such direct connections are those which hold when a belief or a desire, or any other psychological feature, continues to be had.

---

3   *Reasons and Persons*, p. 205. Parfit modifies this definition by adopting Sydney Shoemaker's concept of "Q-memory" to cancel the possible implication that X's remembering Y's experiences already entails by definition that X is the same person as Y (pp. 219-223). I will assume that 'memory' means "Q-memory".

Parfit defines psychological continuity as the ancestral of connectedness. That is, X's being psychologically continuous with Y consists in there being some (possibly empty) series of subjects S1, S2, … such that X is directly connected to S1, who is directly connected to S2, … who is directly connected to Y. Parfit describes this relation between X and Y as consisting in "chains of psychological connectedness", which may overlap.

Initially, Parfit says that what matters in survival is a relation, labeled R, which is a combination of psychological connectedness and continuity. Parfit subsequently qualifies his view, by claiming that some psychological connections are more important than others. The more important connections, he claims, are the ones that involve features that are distinctive of the individual, or features that the individual values in himself.[4]

I suspect that Parfit introduces these qualifications partly because he equivocates on the phrase 'what matters in survival'.[5] Sometimes Parfit interprets the question "What matters in survival?" to mean "Why should one have a first-personal interest in surviving?"[6] Sometimes he takes the question to mean "Why should one have any first-personal concern for the self who will survive?"[7] These two questions exhaust Parfit's ostensible topic, but he obscures this topic with other readings of the question what matters in survival. Sometimes he takes the question to mean "What is it about one's present self whose survival in future selves is worth wanting?"[8] Sometimes he even takes it to mean "What kind of survival is worth wanting?"[9]

The latter readings of the question are not equivalent to the former. One's grounds for taking a first-personal interest in future persons may

---

4   For the importance of a feature's distinctiveness, see pp. 300-301 and note 6 on p. 515. For the importance of a feature's value to the subject, see p. 299. See also the discussion of "The Nineteenth Century Russian" on pp. 327-329.

5   This point was made by Paul Volkening Torek in an unpublished paper and in his Ph.D. dissertation, *Something to look forward to: Personal identity, prudence, and ethics*, University of Michigan, 1995. For the idea that "what matters in survival" is ambiguous in Parfit's usage, see also Tamar Szabó Gendler, "Personal Identity and Thought-Experiments", *The Philosophical Quarterly* 52 (2002), pp. 34-54.

I also suspect that Parfit equivocates on the term 'continuity'. In some contexts, he uses 'continuity' for the ancestral of connectedness. But because he emphasizes the connections that consist in the mere persistence of a trait or attitude, he sometimes understands 'continuity' to mean "qualitative continuity", in the sense that denotes the absence of abrupt qualitative changes. See, e.g., p. 301 of *Reasons and Persons*.

6   See, e.g., p. 260.

7   See, e.g. pp. 282-283.

8   See, e.g., pp. 284, 394, 392.

9   See p. 301.

not depend on their having features of oneself that one has an interest in preserving, or their living lives that one has an interest in living. Conflation of these issues crucially affects Parfit's discussion of problem cases — in particular, the one that he calls the "Branch-Line Case".[10]

In the Branch-Line Case, Parfit imagines a "scanner" that, at the press of a green button, destroys and analyzes his entire body, including his brain. The scanner is linked to a "Replicator" that assembles a molecule-by-molecule copy of him on Mars. He then imagines that the scanner is upgraded to a model that leaves his original body intact, so that there are duplicate versions of him, one on each planet. Finally, he imagines that the upgraded scanner has damaged his heart and that he will consequently die within a few days. Having received this dire prognosis, he speaks with his Replica on Mars by interplanetary videophone:[11]

> Since my Replica knows that I am about to die, he tries to console me with the same thoughts with which I recently tried to console a dying friend. It is sad to learn, on the receiving end, how unconsoling these thoughts are. My Replica then assures me that he will take up my life where I leave off. He loves my wife, and together they will care for my children. And he will finish the book that I am writing. Besides having all of my drafts, he has all of my intentions. I must admit that he can finish my book as well as I could
> ....
>
> If we believe that my Replica is not me, it is natural to assume that my prospect, on the Branch Line, is almost as bad as ordinary death. I shall deny this assumption. As I shall argue later, being destroyed and Replicated is about as good as ordinary survival.

Parfit later explains his view of the case as follows:[12]

> It may be slightly inconvenient that my Replica will be psychologically continuous, not with me as I am now, but with me as I was this morning when I pressed the green button. But these relations are substantially the same. It makes little difference that my life briefly overlaps with that of my Replica.
>
> If the overlap was large, this *would* make a difference. Suppose that I am an old man, who is about to die. I shall be outlived by someone who was once a Replica of me. When this person started to exist forty years ago, he was psychologically continuous with me as I was then. He has since lived

---

10 This case is first introduced on pp. 199-201. It is discussed again on pp. 287-289.

11 p. 201.

12 p. 289.

his own life for forty years. I agree that my relation to *this* Replica, though better than ordinary death, is not nearly as good as ordinary survival. But this relation would be about as good if my Replica would be psychologically continuous with me as I was ten days or ten minutes ago.

Parfit does not explain why the survival of a forty-year-old Replica would be less desirable than that of a Replica produced within the past ten minutes. He seems to imply that the survival of the forty-year-old Replica would be less desirable because he has "lived his own life for forty years" and would be less likely to carry on the life that will be cut short at Parfit's death. At the Replica's creation forty years ago, he might have finished the book that Parfit was writing then, but he now lacks the beliefs, desires, and intentions that would enable him to finish the book that Parfit is writing now and will not survive to finish. Parfit's judgment in this case thus illustrates his view that what matters in survival is the continuation of that in oneself or one's life which one finds important.

Parfit concludes his discussion of the Branch-Line Case with the admission that his judgment is counterintuitive:[13]

> … I admit that this is one of the cases where my view is hardest to believe. *Before* I press the green button, I can more easily believe that my relation to my Replica contains what fundamentally matters in ordinary survival. I can look forward down the Main Line where there are forty years of life ahead. *After* I have pressed the green button, and have talked to my Replica, I cannot in the same way look forward down the Main Line. My concern for the future needs to be redirected. I must try to direct this concern backwards up the Branch Line beyond the point of division, and then forward down the Main Line. This psychological manoeuvre would be difficult. But this is not surprising. And, since it is not surprising, this difficulty does not provide a sufficient argument against what I have claimed about this case.

Parfit's claim, remember, is that although the Replica on the Branch Line will not be meaningfully related to the Original on the Main Line after forty years, the two are meaningfully related, at least for a short while, after the lines diverge.

Of course, none of these considerations come into play in the non-identity problem, which proceeds from the assumption that differences in our environmental policies would lead to the creation of different persons to

---

13 Ibid.

begin with. But I want to consider policies that would be consequential for future generations without greatly affecting their composition.

For example, whether we stockpile nuclear weapons or ban them may someday make the difference between life and death for billions, but unless and until it makes that difference, it may affect the lives of only a few thousands. Across most of the world, the same people will copulate at the same times and under the same conditions irrespective of whether nuclear warheads are lurking on submarines under the sea. And the products of those unions will go on to live the same lives, unless and until the submarines fire their weapons. If the nuclear holocaust occurs in 2150, most of its victims will be the same people as would have been born if we had banned nuclear weapons in 2015. We might therefore think that they will have been harmed by our failure at arms control.

I think otherwise. The sameness of persons across these scenarios would not entail that people in one scenario would have been harmed — not, at least, in the ways that matter, according to Parfit. In order to see why, let's return to Parfit's Branch-Line Case.

When Parfit contemplates that case, in what sense does he find himself directing his concern "up" one line and "down" the other? Clearly, 'up' and 'down' in this case represent the direction of time. Parfit later says that psychological continuity is a transitive relation in either temporal direction but not "if we allow it to take both directions in a single argument".[14] That is, the reason why Parfit is not psychologically continuous with any of his Replicas is that the psychological connections between them run first backward in time, up to the point of division, and then forward, down the "Main Line". But why should this change of temporal direction make any difference? Parfit doesn't say. He simply admits that when directing his self-concern through time, he has difficulty switching directions.

I suggest that concern for his "Main Line" Replica is difficult for Branch-Line Parfit because the direction of time is also the direction of causation, which is the direction in which information can be conveyed. The change of direction severs internal communication between Parfit and his Replica, in the sense that their psychological connections cannot carry information between them. Parfit's conception of psychological connections has all along implied that they are channels of information, but he has chosen

---

14 p. 302.

instead to emphasize the relations of resemblance between their input and output — between experiences and the corresponding memories, intentions and the corresponding actions, psychological features and their subsequent instantiation — rather than the fact that these inputs and outputs are connected in ways that convey information.[15] Yet Parfit's difficulty in feeling concern for his Replica seems to indicate that internal communication with earlier or later selves is significant.

I now turn to an explanation of why such communication is significant. After that, I will return to the non-identity problem.

Selfhood in Dreams

Last night I dreamed that I was Wittgenstein brandishing a poker at Karl Popper. (I am prone to nightmares.)[16]

---

15 See pp. 286-287, where Parfit discusses the case in which psychological continuity and connectedness have a cause that isn't reliable. Parfit says that a Replica to whom one is unreliably connected is just as good as one to whom one's connection is reliable. He compares this case to that of a medication that effects a cure sometimes but not reliably: "This effect is just as good, even though its cause was unreliable." This analogy suggests that what matters in survival are the effects of one's causal connections to future selves, not the connections themselves.

16 This and the next several sections draw on material from my "Self to Self", *The Philosophical Review* 105 (1996): 39-76; reprinted in *Self to Self: Selected Essays* (Cambridge: Cambridge University Press, 2005), pp. 170-202. That paper draws in turn on Bernard Williams's "Imagination and the Self", in *Problems of the Self: Philosophical Papers 1956– 1972* (Cambridge: Cambridge University Press, 1973), pp. 26-45. Parfit makes a similar point on p. 221:

> Since Jane seems to remember *seeing* the lightning, she seems to remember *herself* seeing the lightning. Her apparent memory may tell her accurately what Paul's experience was like, but it tells her, falsely, that it was *she* who had this experience.
>
> There may be a sense in which this claim is true. Jane's apparent memories may come to her in what [Christopher] Peacocke calls *the first-person mode of presentation*. Thus, when she seems to remember walking across the Piazza, she might seem to remember seeing a child running *towards her*. If this is what she seems to remember, she must be seeming to remember *herself* seeing this child running towards her.
>
> We might deny these claims. In a dream, I can seem to see myself from a point of view *outside* my own body. I might seem to see myself running towards that point of view. Since it is *myself* that I seem to see running in this direction, this direction cannot be towards *myself*. I might say that I seem to see myself running towards *the seer's point of view*. And this could be said to be the direction in which Jane seems to remember seeing this child run. So described, Jane's apparent memory would include no references to herself.
>
> Though we could deny that Jane's apparent memories must seem, in part, to be about herself, there is no need to do so. Even if her apparent memories are presented in the first-person mode, Jane need not assume that, if they are not delusions, they must be memories of her *own* experiences….

Now, when I say, "I dreamed that I was Wittgenstein," my first use of 'I', in "I dreamed", refers to me, David Velleman, who groaned in his sleep and then woke up remembering a nightmare. What about my second use of 'I', the one in "I was Wittgenstein"? That use of 'I' occurs within a that-clause reporting the content of my dream. That is, I had a dream with the content "I am Ludwig Wittgenstein brandishing a poker at Karl Popper." I might even have included this content in the dream itself, since I might have dreamed of declaring, "Here am I, brandishing a poker at Karl Popper!" The reference that 'I' would have had within the dream itself ("Here am *I*...") determines the reference of 'I' in my dream-report ("... dreamed that *I* was..."). To whom would the first 'I' have referred?

I didn't dream that David Velleman was Wittgenstein. While dreaming, I was temporarily oblivious to the existence of David Velleman — oblivious, in fact, to my own actual existence under any name or description whatsoever.[17] Had I dreamed of saying "Here am I", the pronoun 'I' would have referred to the speaker of those words, and the speaker of those words would have been, not the actual David Velleman, but the dreamed-of Ludwig Wittgenstein. Indeed, I could have dreamed of saying, "Here am I, Ludwig Wittgenstein, brandishing a poker!"

Yet I couldn't report the dream by saying, "I dreamed that Ludwig Wittgenstein was Ludwig Wittgenstein brandishing a poker at Karl Popper." In "I dreamed that I was Wittgenstein," the second 'I' *refers* to Wittgenstein, but it can't be replaced by an expression that refers to him *as* Wittgenstein. And of course it doesn't refer to me, David Velleman. What accounts for the use of 'I' in my dream-report?

What accounts for it is that the dream was about Wittgenstein from the first-personal point of view. In the dream, everything was represented from Wittgenstein's perspective. The meaning rule for the pronoun 'I' is that it refers to the speaker, who is the subject of the perspective from which the pronoun is spoken. The dream represented everything from Wittgenstein's perspective, and the pronoun 'I' spoken from the same perspective would have referred to Wittgenstein. And when I, David Velleman, report the content of the dream, I refer to Wittgenstein as 'I' in order to indicate that the dream was from his perspective — that he (and not Popper, for example) was the "I" in the context of the dream.

---

17 For help with this analysis of first-person reference in dreams, I am indebted to Imogen Dickie.

Selfhood in Memories

Now consider a veridical memory: I can remember when my grandfather took me to the Empire State Building as a child. To whom does 'me' refer in this memory-report?

Of course, you will say that 'me' refers to David Velleman. But at the moment, that answer begs the question, since we are trying to evaluate theories of personal identity, which aim to explain how one and the same person, David Velleman, could have a six-year-old self in 1958 and a sixty-two-year-old self today — or, in other words, how that six-year-old and this sixty-two-year-old could belong to one and the same person. Conveniently for us, the six-year-old went by the name of Jamie. So we can ask our question like this: When I say, "I remember when my grandfather took me to the Empire State Building", does 'me' refer to David or to Jamie?

Obviously, it isn't a sixty-two-year old who appears with his grandfather in my memory. In my memory, my grandfather (he was called Chick) is taking a six-year-old to the Empire State Building — the six-year-old named Jamie. But if I say that I remember when Chick took *Jamie* to the Empire State Building, I would leave out the bit about Jamie's being *me*. My memory isn't about Chick taking some six-year-old to the Empire State Building and calling him Jamie. I remember him taking the six-year-old *me*. But of course the expression 'the six-year-old me' describes the very phenomenon that we're trying to understand. How could a six-year-old have been a past self of this sixty-two-year-old; how could *he* have been *me*?

One answer would be that my memory simply contains the thought that the character in my memory was me, the one having the memory — as if in having the memory, I point to the six-year-old and think "That's me." Another answer would be that my memory is accompanied by the thought that it *is* a memory, meaning that it represents an experience that I, the rememberer, once had — as if in having the memory, I think, "Here's an experience from my past."

Neither of these answers seems satisfactory. I can have a memory without realizing that it *is* a memory, and yet it can still be about the time when my grandfather took me to the Empire State Building. And if I remembered instead a time when my grandfather took my whole kindergarten to the Empire State Building, I could mentally point to any one of the children and think "That's me," but that's not the sense in which I do in fact remember that my grandfather took me.

I propose that the sense in which I remember that he took me is the same as the sense in which I dreamed that I was Wittgenstein. The memory represents things from the perspective of the child being taken to the Empire State Building. I have a memory from a perspective in which 'me' would refer to Jamie — a perspective in which Jamie was "me". In the context of my dream, "I" was Wittgenstein; in the context of my memory, Jamie is "me".

Here is a difference between the memory and the dream. The memory gets to be "of" or about me in a different way from that in which the dream was "of" or about Wittgenstein.

The perceptual experiences that made up my dream — the sights and sounds — didn't pick out Wittgenstein and Popper as the people involved. They were just perceptual experience from the perspective someone or other, as brandishing a poker at someone or other. In what sense, then, was it a dream about Wittgenstein and Popper? The dream-experiences must have been somehow accompanied by the thought "Wittgenstein brandishing a poker at Popper".[18] In this respect, a dream is like a game of make-believe. I can pretend to be Wittgenstein brandishing a poker at Popper, but I can't do it just by waving a poker at you. I have to say, "Let's pretend I'm Wittgenstein …" or something of the sort. I have to *stipulate* who "I" am in the make-believe; similarly, there must have been some silent thought stipulating who "I" was in my dream.

Not so with a memory. My memory is about Jamie without stipulation. Why? Because the memory is a record of an experience, and the experience was Jamie's, hence a context in which Jamie was "me". If Jamie had taken a photograph with his Brownie camera, it would have been an image of the Empire State Building as photographed by his camera. If I retrieved that picture from my album and scanned it into my computer, the image on my screen would also be an image of the Empire State Building as photographed by Jamie's camera. Similarly, Jamie's visual experience and its traces in my visual memory are both images of the Empire State Building as seen by Jamie. He and I don't need to accompany those images with the thought "Empire State Building as seen by Jamie". That's what the images are, whether we think so or not.

---

18 The thought "I am Wittgenstein", as entertained by the "I" of the dream, would not have been sufficient, since it would have been compatible with the dream's being about a madman who thought he was Wittgenstein.

So whereas the visual images in my dream are about Wittgenstein only by courtesy of some stipulating thought, the visual images of my memory are really about Jamie, because he experienced them and I am retrieving traces of them. Consequently, Wittgenstein can't be the "I" of my dream unless I know who he was, so that I can (while dreaming) have a thought specifying him as the one whose experiences I am dreaming. But Jamie can be the "I" of my memories even if I have no idea who he was — even if I have amnesia about my so-called "identity". Jamie can be the "I" of my memories so long as he is the one whose experiences I am remembering, in the sense that I am retrieving traces of them from memory.

Here is another way to put the contrast. I can dream of Wittgenstein in the first person, but only by picking him out in the third person, so as to specify (while dreaming) that he is the "I" of my dream. By contrast, I can remember Jamie in the first person without any further thought, simply because my memory is a context in which he really is "me". You might say, I'm on first-personal terms with Jamie. To be on a "first-name basis" with someone is to be in a position to call him by his first name without being introduced; to be on a first-person basis is to be in a position to refer to him in the first person without stipulation.

I suggest that the psychological connections that matter for personal survival are connections of genuine first-person reference — connections of the sort that enable me to think about Jamie in the first person without further thought. I can think about him as "me" simply because I have first-personal thoughts that are "of" him in actual fact.

The relevant connections are causal. Like photographs, experiences are "of" whatever they are received from, and their copies are of the same things by virtue of the causal process of copying. Note, in fact, that causation is more important than resemblance. After scanning a photograph into my computer, I can apply all sorts of visual effects to it without changing what it is an image of. A distorted image of the Empire State Building is still an image of the Empire State Building. Similarly, a faulty memory of the Empire State Building can still be a memory of the Empire State Building, provided that it is causally derived from an experience (even a distorted experience) of the Empire State Building.

Here, then, is a clue to the flaw in Parfit's reasoning about the Branch-Line Case. Shortly after the branch in the road, Parfit and his Replica are psychologically very similar, having inherited the same memories, beliefs, desires, plans, and traits from their common predecessor. But Parfit and his Replica are not causally connected with one another: neither one can inherit traces of the other's experiences, and so neither can be the "I" in the other's thoughts. In short, they aren't on first-personal terms. Hence they aren't connected in the way that matters for personal survival.

Selfhood in Anticipation

Consider now a different connection that conducts first-person reference through time. I think I'll take my grandchildren to the Empire State Building. I have grandchildren, and I'm going to take them to the places where my grandfather took me (with some regrettable exceptions, like the old Yankee Stadium). Here I am referring to a particular future grandfather. We need a name for him, so that we can ask what makes him my future self. My eldest grandchild calls me Boppa, so let's give the name 'Boppa' to the future grandfather who will take his grandchildren to the Empire State Building, among other landmarks.

I may be forming a plan — that is, a thought designed to initiate the outing that it represents. Alternatively, I may simply be predicting rather than planning the outing. If I'm predicting it, however, I am not merely predicting it; I'm predicting it with a feeling of anticipatory excitement. In either case, my thought is one that can be resolved, or given closure, by the outing that it represents — resolved or given closure either when my plan is carried out or when the associated excitement is discharged.

The reason why my present thought can be resolved in the future is that it will be stored in my memory, ready to reemerge in Boppa's consciousness at a later date, when its sense of determination or expectancy can be discharged by the corresponding action or experience. Boppa will find himself with the thought "I am going to take my grandchildren to the Empire State Building," and he will be in a position to see it through to its practical or experiential fulfillment by interpreting the first-person pronoun without any further thought — hence as referring to him. Indeed, my present thought includes this future resolution of itself. It represents a future outing as implementing or verifying this very thought as retrieved from memory.[19] So when Boppa interprets the first-person pronoun as

---

19 See Maurice Merleau-Ponty, *Phenomenology of Perception*: "[W]ith my immediate past, I have also the horizon of futurity which surrounded it, and thus I have my actual present seen as the future of that past. With the imminent future, I have the horizon of past which

referring to him, he will be interpreting the pronoun as was intended when the thought was formed. I don't mean that the pronoun was intended to refer to Boppa; I mean that it was intended to refer to whoever would retrieve the thought from memory and then be in a position to interpret the pronoun, without further stipulation, as referring to him.

In this respect, my thought is like a message in a bottle.

Suppose that I am stranded on a desert island and I launch a bottle containing a note that says, "If you find this message and bring it to my wife in New York, she will reward you with $10,000." To whom does 'you' refer in the context of my note? It refers to whoever finds the note. (If the note is never found, my use of 'you' fails to refer.) Alone on my desert island, I have no one to whom I can refer in the second person — no one with whom I am, so to speak, on second-personal terms. In casting my message on the waters, I am hoping to *get* onto second-personal terms with someone, by succeeding in my attempt to refer with the pronoun 'you'. That referential hope is part and parcel of my hope to communicate with someone by way of the message.

So it is with my thought of a future outing. I represent the outing as taken by someone who has retrieved this very thought and can resolve it without any further thought about who is meant by 'I'. I hope that there will be a subject to take himself without further thought as the "I" in the context, just as I hope that there will be a reader to intercept the second-personal reference in my message. If my hope for the thought is fulfilled, I will have succeeded in thinking with it about a future subject in the first person. What I am hoping, then, is to get onto first-personal terms with someone in the future, someone who will fulfill my present intention or expectation.

The case of my future-directed thoughts goes beyond this analogy in one important respect. Just as I can frame a first-personal thought that Boppa will be able to interpret in the future as referring to him, he will be able to think first-personally about having himself formed that thought in the past. That is, he will be able to think "I planned ..." or "I expected ..." and thereby think of me without stipulating that I am who he means by 'I'. He will therefore fulfill an intention or resolve an emotion that he conceives

---

will surround it, and therefore my actual present as the past of that future" (*Maurice Merleau-Ponty: Basic Writings*, ed. Thomas Baldwin [London: Routledge, 2003], p. 82).

as having belonged to himself — that is, to someone with whom he is on first-personal terms.

Selfhood in Other Possible Worlds

What matters in survival, I suggest, is being able to think about the future as resolving this very thought. What matters is being able to have thoughts that aren't closed off in the sense of being barred future closure. Of course, I care whether the future will answer my thoughts in the sense of bearing them out, by making them come true. But I care even more, and more fundamentally, whether my thoughts will be answered in the sense that future actions or experiences will be *felt* as fulfilling them, as if concluding a musical call-and-response. I don't just care that my hopes will be fulfilled; I care that they will survive to be discharged in a sense of gratification. I don't just care that my fears will not be realized; I care that they will be allayed or relieved.

I also care about communicating on first-personal terms with the subjects of those experiences. I think about their life "from the inside" not just by thinking about it from their point of view but also by conceiving of that point of view as one in which this very thought will emerge from memory, so that the thought itself will be "inside" the anticipated experiences, and my present self will be internally accessible to their subjects as "me". My thought therefore presents itself as inside the point of view from which it represents future events.

This inside view of their experiences has an intimacy that I value. One important aspect of intimacy is the ability to dispense with referential cues. We recognize long-married couples, for example, by their telegraphic style of conversation, in which they use pronouns without antecedents — without even following one another's gaze — because of already knowing what is salient to one another. Similarly, I can think of a future self as "me" and rely on him to know that I meant *him* — that is, the self to whom he will naturally attach the reference.[20] Because referential cues are the means of coordinating different points of view, doing without them gives the impression of occupying a single point of view. Like a long-married couple, then, I and my future self seem to share a single point of view because of being referentially in sync.

---

20 This intimacy would be lacking if I were going to undergo fission, as in the Branch-Line Case. I discuss this issue in "Self to Self".

If I am right about what matters in survival, then the relevant aspect of psychological connectedness is not the one that interests Parfit. What interests Parfit, as we have seen, is the relation of resemblance between the termini of psychological connections: the experiences and their corresponding memories, the intentions and the corresponding actions, the acquired attitudes or traits and their persisting instantiation. These psychological causes and effects often perpetuate various features of mine, and Parfit believes that those features which are distinctive of me, or valuable to me, count more than others in constituting what matters in survival. As I have argued, however, the aspect of psychological connectedness that really counts is the causal relation that establishes an informational channel to carry anticipations forward to their anticipated cadences, and to carry future-directed references forward to find their referents, including the future "me". Whether the same connections preserve any of my features is relatively unimportant.

My account of what matters in survival thus explains why Parfit has difficulty caring first-personally about his Replica in the Branch-Line Case. He can neither store thoughts to be retrieved by his Replica nor retrieve thoughts that are stored by him, and so he can neither experience his future as responding to the Replica's thoughts nor expect the Replica's future to be experienced as responding to his. The causal tides can carry no internal messages between them. Even if the Replica finishes Parfit's current book-project, its completion will not discharge the hopes that Parfit has now, on the Branch Line, and so Parfit can no longer aim his hopes at such an experienced fulfillment. As far as he is concerned, his book will be finished by someone else — someone who is like him, perhaps, but who is not himself, because of being in no position to complete the phrases of his current mental life.

I thus arrive at the conclusion that Parfit's difficulty in caring first-personally about a Replica is unsurprising for reasons that do not deprive the difficulty of philosophical significance. On the contrary, his difficulty in caring first-personally about his Replica is unsurprising for the very good reason that he and his Replica are not on first-personal terms.

My conclusion has implications that reach beyond the realm of science fiction. A person's Replicas are not the only candidate selves from whom he is causally isolated in a way that blocks internal communication, thus preventing them from being his selves in fact. Also causally isolated from the person are his other possible selves — himself as he or his life might have been. I will describe this merely possible person as himself in other possible worlds.

Before embarking on this topic, I will need to regiment my language carefully. From now on, I will use the term 'selves' for those subjects who are connected to me by the relation that conveys first-personal concern. Since the present question is whether inhabitants of other possible worlds can bear that relation to me, it amounts to the question whether I have other possible selves at all. The candidates for selfhood in this case are inhabitants of other possible worlds who are numerically identical to the person I am — that is, to David Velleman. I am not questioning whether David Velleman exists in other possible worlds: I think he does. What I am questioning is whether David Velleman as he might have been is any self of mine.[21]

But what shall we call him in relation to me? We can't refer to him as another possible self, since his selfhood with me is the relation that is currently in question. I propose that we call him my identical.

I often wonder what would have become of me if I hadn't decided to go back to graduate school in 1978. Maybe I would have become a freelance writer. There are possible worlds in which I did become a freelance writer: in some of them I am living just a few blocks from where I live today. I wonder whether I have children in those worlds. And so on.

The James David Velleman living in those worlds diverged from my actual path in 1978, and since then he has followed a very different path from mine. My relation to this identical is therefore similar to Parfit's relation to his Replica in the Branch-Line Case. In order for my concern to reach the other possible David Velleman, it would have to travel "backwards up the Branch Line", rewinding my years as a philosopher, back to the moment of my decision to go to graduate school, "and then forward down the Main Line", playing out the life I would have lived if I had decided to become a writer instead. In my view, this maneuver cannot convey genuine self-concern, because it does not follow a possible channel of information

---

21 In considering this question, I needn't worry about the metaphysical dispute between counterpart theorists and theorists who posit strict transworld identities. Whether another possible David Velleman is related to me in the way that justifies self-concern doesn't depend on whether he is strictly identical to me or merely more similar to me than anyone else in his world. (I do wonder, however, whether the inaccessibility of transworld identicals to self-concern played a role in David Lewis's intuitions when he developed his counterpart theory.)

between me and its object, and so it cannot direct my concern to someone meaningfully conceived of as "me".

In short, my relation to the person I would have been in another possible world does not include what matters in survival. Although I am the same person as the David Velleman who became a freelance writer, he is not a self of mine in the sense that calls for me to identify with him, or to identify my interests with his. He and I may be numerically identical, but — as Parfit himself puts it — identity is not what matters.[22]

Back in 1978, of course, I was in a position to look down many alternative paths and to form first-personal thoughts that would have succeeded in picking out the traveler on any one of them, had he been the one to end up carrying the traces of those thoughts, available for later retrieval from memory. Looking forward, then, I could have entertained self-concern for many different possible future selves, concern that might in each case have turned out to be about a future person.

After the point of decision, however, alternative paths were closed to me not only in practice but also in first-personal thought. Whatever befalls the travelers on those paths is what would have befallen David Velleman, if I had decided differently, but his being David Velleman is, so to speak, nothing to me: it doesn't matter in the same way as my being the one who might undergo different fates in the future, depending on what I now decide.

The Irrationality of Grudges and Regret

Here is a reason for not regretting what might have been — a reason other than the ordinary, pragmatic reason that nothing can be done about it. It is not just practically useless to have regrets about what might have been; it's metaphysically confused, because the world as it might have been does not include anyone for whom I can have first-personal concern. I can perhaps envy the people for whom things might have gone differently, as I envy

---

22 Thanks to Elena Weinstein for making this connection. As Matt Hanser has pointed out to me, this conception of what matters in survival helps to explain why, as Lucretius observed, we want to die later but don't regret not having been born earlier. We cannot complete psychological cadences for the past selves who would have been born earlier, but we can start psychological cadences for our longer-lived future selves to complete. Some explain the difference by arguing that we would not have been identical with a person born earlier. (See Thomas Nagel, "Death", in *Mortal Questions* [New York: Cambridge University Press, 1991], pp. 4-10.) I think that the explanation does not depend on the necessity of our origins. Even if we could have been identical with an earlier-born person, our relation to that person lacks what matters in survival.

any other person. But I cannot think of them as my more fortunate selves, because they aren't selves of mine in the relevant sense, and so I cannot regard what they have as something that I myself might have had.

At issue here is only a particular kind of regret, namely, regret about what might have been. Another kind of regret, often called agent-regret, is about what my actual selves did in the past. There is no confusion in regret over past mistakes, since I am first-personally related to the agents who made them. The confusion begins when I regret not having today what I might have had if I hadn't made those mistakes back then.

The person who might have been better off today if I had done differently in the past — that person is inaccessible to my self-concern. Of course he is who I might have been — that is, who could have been a future self of my past self, because he is on first-personal terms with someone with whom I am still on first-personal terms. But as it turns out, selfhood is not transitive: another future self of my past self is not a self of mine. The fate of a merely possible self of mine is no more pertinent to me than anyone else's, since I can only imagine undergoing that fate.

Thus, I shouldn't regret not having what I could have had, because no self of mine could have had it. I can rationally *envy* the David Velleman who could have had what I don't. I can also rationally gloat over what I have that he wouldn't have. Envy and gloating are appropriate with respect to others. But regret is a first-personal emotion, and what I could have had could have been had only by someone with whom I am not on first-personal terms.

But suppose that someone stole my identity and emptied my bank account. I am now reduced to poverty, daydreaming about the comfortable life I would have had if only my passwords had been longer. Surely, the thief harmed me, and we are tempted to say that the harm consists precisely in my being poorer than I might have been. But according to my view, it seems, I have no grounds for resenting the harm, because I am not first-personally related to the David Velleman who would have been better off.

My view still leaves me grounds for resentment, however — namely, that the thief harmed my past self by depriving him of a comfortable future. When I complain, "I could have been better off," I don't mean, "I have a better-off possible self"; I mean, "I (in the past) had the chance of being better off in the future."

The moral upshot is that resentment should wane as time passes. If, on the contrary, my resentment should be proportional to the difference between my present actual self and other present possible David Vellemans, then it should increase as time passes, since those other David Vellemans would have had capital to invest and I didn't. The difference between our financial circumstances has therefore grown over time, and so should my resentment, if rational resentment is proportional to the difference between contemporaneous possible David Vellemans. But rational resentment is rather vicarious resentment on behalf of my past self, who recedes further and further into the past, hence further and further from my first-personal concern. In short, rationality favors letting bygones be bygones, in proportion to how far bygone they are.

The Identity Problem

An extension of this reasoning leads to the conclusion that I cannot rationally resent past actions that were taken before I was born. Resentment of past actions must be based on their having deprived my past selves of something they might have had, including possible futures. But the David Vellemans born in possible worlds that had already diverged from ours are merely my identicals, not my selves, since there is no possible channel of internal communication between us. And I don't have any prenatal selves who might have looked forward to alternative futures consisting of my actual life and the lives of those counterfactual David Vellemans. So I have no past selves who were deprived of those futures. In sum, I am not on first-personal terms with anyone who could have been deprived of anything by actions taken before I was born.

Non-identity is thus inessential to Parfit's problem. Recall that the non-identity problem is how our wasting resources today can harm people who will be born in the future, given that our conserving resources would have prevented those people from being born. The people who will inherit a depleted Earth from us wouldn't have been born to enjoy the plentiful Earth that we might have left behind us instead. How, asks Parfit, will they have been harmed by their inferior inheritance?

But it now turns out that even if the people who inherit the depleted Earth would still have been born to enjoy the plentiful one, they will have no complaint against us on self-regarding grounds, since they will have no first-personal relationship to their counterfactual counterparts. They will be no worse off than they might have been, because the people who would have been better off are their mere identicals, not their selves.

Parfit thinks that the non-identity problem raises a moral objection to evaluating the effect of our actions on future generations in what he calls person-affecting terms — that is, in terms of whether our actions today will make future persons better or worse off than those same persons would otherwise have been. The moral objection to person-affecting evaluation is that it yields the morally unacceptable conclusion that we cannot harm future generations by depleting the Earth's resources, polluting the environment, wrecking just institutions, or doing anything else that would cause different people to be born.

I have argued that person-affecting evaluation is not only morally unacceptable but metaphysically confused, and that it is confused even with respect to courses of action that would not affect who is born. People simply cannot be harmed or benefitted by actions taken before their births. The circumstances into which they are born, including the range of their possible futures, cannot make them better or worse off than anyone first-personally related to them would have been; nor, of course, do they have any past selves who could have been harmed or benefitted in that way. People's initial endowments at birth are the baseline against which all harms and benefits to them must be assessed.

Parfit thinks that the alternative to person-affecting evaluation is to evaluate our effect on future people in terms of the average or total welfare they would enjoy, irrespective of who they would be. Unfortunately, those methods of evaluation lead to other morally unacceptable conclusions. The result seems to be a stalemate between methods of evaluation, none of which we can accept.

The way out of the stalemate, of course, is to abjure consequentialist evaluation of any kind. The right way to think about our obligations to future generations is to think, not about providing for their well-being, but about respecting their humanity, an approach that does not take account of who or how many they are. I will develop this approach in Parts II and III of this series.

II. The Gift of Life[23]

They will arrange for the suckling of the children by bringing their mothers to the nursery when their breasts are still full, taking every precaution to see that no mother recognizes her child.

—Plato, *Republic* V.ii.460e

Nor is there any way of preventing brothers and children and fathers and mothers from sometimes recognizing one another; for children are born like their parents, and they will necessarily be finding indications of their relationship to one another.

—Aristotle, *Politics* II.iii.1262a

Many people are grateful to their parents for giving them a gift consisting in life itself. Life itself is an odd sort of gift, since there is no one around antecedently to serve as its intended recipient.[24] Life is at best a benefit that prospective parents toss into the void in the hope that someone will turn out to have snagged it, to his own surprise as much as anyone's. But once parents have performed this random act of kindness, they may be thought to have no further obligation to the future beneficiary, for whom they have already done more than anyone will ever again be able to do.

Of course, babies are needy creatures, and their biological parents generally bear the burden of seeing to it that their needs are met. This allocation of childcare duties may be no more than a social convenience, however, taking advantage of the biological fact that at least one of the parents is bound to be on the scene when the needy creature makes its appearance. Maybe alternative childcare arrangements would be just as good, if only they could be institutionalized, as Plato famously imagined. If proximity to the birth is all that biological parents have going for them as caregivers, Plato's scheme for community nurseries may be worth considering.

---

23 This part was presented to the Legal Theory Working Group at The Baldy Center for Law & Social Policy, University of Buffalo, and to the Legal Theory Workshop at the University of Toronto Faculty of Law. I also had helpful discussions or correspondence on the topic with Jules Coleman, Daniela Dover, Robin Jeshion, Arthur Ripstein, Brian Slattery, and Paul F. Velleman.

24 As Matthew Hanser pointed out, no one can act with the intention of bringing a particular person into existence ("Harming Future People", *Philosophy & Public Affairs* 19 [1990]: 47-70, p. 61).

Aristotle criticized this scheme as unrealistic. Children who are not seen as the sons and daughters of anyone in particular will not be properly cared for, he thought; and in any case, people will seek out their own parents, children, and siblings, despite all efforts to keep them apart. As Aristotle realized, human beings have a natural tendency to find and associate with their biological relatives.

Today we can explain this tendency in evolutionary terms, since it enables each human organism to promote the propagation of his genotype and to benefit from the like tendency of his relatives. But the aims of natural selection need not be ours. If the human tendency to congregate in biological families is a vestige of natural selection, then it may be like the capacity for murderous jealousy, for example — a natural tendency that human society has no reason to accommodate. Certainly, the human affinity for consanguines is implicated in such regrettable human phenomena as racism and xenophobia. Maybe it should be killed in the cradle, as Plato suggested.

Still, that's not what modern-day readers of *The Republic* think; they think that Plato's scheme for child rearing is inhumane. Why do they think so? What would be wrong with permanently separating parents and children at birth?

I think that associating with relatives is more than a biological imperative; it's a personal need, imposed on persons like us by our predicament as human beings. Because I believe that biological ties have value, I also believe that there are good reasons for assigning the duties of child-rearing to biological parents in the first instance. Indeed, I believe that the act of procreation generates parental obligations that cannot be contracted out to others, except when doing so is in the best interests of the child.[25]

These obligations arise because being begotten is not, as many believe, the original birthday present. As Seana Shiffrin has argued in a brilliant paper on claims of wrongful life, being brought into existence is at best a mixed blessing, and those who confer it are not entitled to walk away congratulating themselves on a job well done.[26]

---

25 For a different defense of the same position, see Rivka Weinberg, "The Moral Complexity of Sperm Donation", *Bioethics* 22 (2008): 166-178.

26 Seana Valentine Shiffrin, "Wrongful Life, Procreative Responsibility, and the Significance of Harm", *Legal Theory* 5 (1999): 117-148. Brad Inwood has directed me to Seneca's *De Beneficiis*, Book 3, Sections 29-38. For example: "[I]t is a pretty trivial benefit for a father and mother to sleep together unless there are additional benefits to follow up on this

Shiffrin argues that bringing someone into existence is a morally equivocal act, because it entails imposing harms on the person as well as bestowing benefits. Shiffrin argues further that a fundamental asymmetry between harms and benefits prevents the harm imposed by procreation from being justified by the benefit bestowed. And Shiffrin attempts to explain the asymmetry by proposing a philosophical account of harm, although she does not develop it fully.[27]

Now, although I agree with Shiffrin that bringing someone into existence is a morally equivocal act, I do not think that it can be equivocal because of conferring a mixture of harms and benefits. For as I explained in Part I, I believe that a person can be neither harmed nor benefited by being brought into existence. I will therefore devote the first half of this part to paraphrasing Shiffrin's arguments in slightly different terms, by drawing out elements, already implicit in them, of an Aristotelian conception of human well-being. I will then draw some conclusions that are congruent with Shiffrin's and a few more that I doubt whether she would endorse.

The best way to explain Shiffrin's conception of harm, I think, is to apply it, not to cases of harm per se, but to the philosophical problem of distinguishing between pain and suffering. That pain and suffering are distinct is obvious from the many cases of pain that do not occasion suffering (stubbed toes, skinned knees), as well as cases of suffering that do not necessarily involve pain (loneliness, boredom).

What makes the difference between pain and suffering is *coping*. Suffering occurs when someone cannot or does not cope with adversity of some kind. To cope with pain or other adversity is to exercise, or to give oneself the sense of exercising, some degree of control over the adversity itself or, at least, over one's reactions to it. Coping is therefore a way of exercising one's will in the face of adverse circumstances, by managing one's response to them and maybe also by managing the circumstances themselves.

---

initial gift and to consolidate it with additional services to the child. It is not living which is the good, but living well. And I do live well. But I could have lived badly" (Section 38, Inwood's translation).

27 That the goods and ills of existence are in some sense asymmetric is an intuition discussed by several philosophers. See, e.g., Trudy Govier, "What Should We Do About Future People?", *American Philosophical Quarterly* 16 (1979): 105-113; David Benatar, "Why It Is Better Never to Come Into Existence", *American Philosophical Quarterly* 34 (1997): 345-355; and Michael Tooley, "Value, Obligation and the Asymmetry Question", *Bioethics* 12 (1998): 111-124. The issue is also discussed by Derek Parfit, *Reasons and Persons*, p. 391.

When someone fails to cope, we describe him as going to pieces, falling apart, breaking down — all expressions that reflect damage not just to the body or to personal projects but to the self.[28] Failure to cope entails damage to the self because it entails a defeat or disabling of the will. The person is thrown into a condition of helplessness in the face of some obstacle or assault. Stripped of his agency, he is damaged in his very personhood. The fact and the experience of this damage to the self are constitutive of suffering.[29]

This brief account of suffering echoes Shiffrin's account of harm. She suggests that harm consists in a condition toward which a person finds himself in a position of passive subjection — the position, as Shiffrin puts it, of an "endurer". She thus reverses the order of explanation between the badness of harm and our unwillingness to undergo it. It's not that we're unwilling to undergo something harmful because it's bad; rather, something is bad enough to qualify as harmful if and because we find ourselves undergoing it unwillingly.

Shiffrin also briefly suggests a corresponding account of benefit. What she says is that unsought benefits are not as good as benefits that the recipient has chosen to pursue and has succeeded in obtaining. She thereby suggests that, while being passively withstood is constitutive of harm, being actively sought and attained is at least characteristic of benefit.

These remarks about harm and benefit ground Shiffrin's explanation of the asymmetry between the harms and benefits entailed in the gift of life. In Shiffrin's view, the asymmetry arises from the fact that the gift of life is never sought or even accepted by its recipient. He simply becomes aware, long after the fact, of having been stuck with it. Even if the recipient welcomes this gift retrospectively, his will was nevertheless preempted when it was given to him, since he had no chance to refuse or accept. The harms that accompany this gift are consequently aggravated by having been imposed on him willy-nilly, with the result that he is already in a relation of passive subjection to them from the start. And the associated

---

28 For this account of suffering, see Eric J. Cassell, "Recognizing Suffering", *The Hastings Center Report* 21 (1991): 24-31. See also Kathy Charmaz, "Loss of Self: A Fundamental Form of Suffering in the Chronically Ill", *Sociology of Health & Illness* 5 (1983): 168-195.

29 Because coping is an exercise of the will, it requires choice on the part of the subject. That's why we can sometimes think that people have chosen to suffer, although we're never quite sure. There is no clear line between inability and unwillingness to cope, but there certainly are cases in which someone could cope but chooses not to; or maybe he cannot choose to cope.

benefits are somewhat undermined by lacking the features of choice and successful effort that belong to the most significant benefits.

Thus Shiffrin. Much as I admire her attempt to explain the asymmetry between the goods and ills of existence, I do not believe that a balance of goods and ills can account for what is morally equivocal about procreation. Still, I think that her explanation points us in the right direction, by pointing us toward an Aristotelian conception of human well-being.

According to Aristotle, human well-being consists in the exercise of capacities that are in excellent condition, and pleasure is that complete absorption in the exercise of one's capacities which their being in excellent condition tends to facilitate.[30] The excellent condition of one's capacities is what Aristotle called *aretê*. His claim that pleasure consists in being absorbed or engrossed in exercising one's capacities has been confirmed by research into what psychologists call "flow".[31]

Aristotle's conceptions of well-being and pleasure are hospitable to Shiffrin's account of harm and its asymmetrical relation to benefit. Anything that casts a person into a state of passive subjection will prevent him from exercising his capacities, and it will also deprive him of the enjoyment of becoming absorbed in their exercise. Conversely, any good that is acquired through the exercise of the relevant capacities will bring with it a bonus of flourishing and "flow", like a destination that lies at the end of an engrossing journey.

I think that Aristotle's conceptions of human well-being and pleasure also carry implications for the value of the so-called gift of life, because they imply that human happiness *takes work*. It takes work in the form of exercising one's proper capacities; more importantly, it takes work because the relevant capacities must be acquired by practice and habituation. In this respect, humans are unlike other animals, whose well-being consists mostly in the exercise of capacities that are innate. A cat is born already equipped for the activities that will constitute its flourishing; a human being must be educated and trained for his most rewarding activities.

---

30 'Well-being' and 'flourishing' are not precise equivalents for Aristotle's 'eudaimonia', since they can be achieved at a particular time, whereas eudaimonia can be achieved only over the course of an entire life.

31 Mihaly Csikszentmihalyi, *Flow: The Psychology of Optimal Experience* (New York: Harper & Row, 1990).

According to the Aristotelian view, then, a human child is born with the general, second-order capacity to acquire the further, specific capacities whose exercise will eventually constitute its flourishing as an adult. The gift of life is therefore the gift of an opportunity — the opportunity to do the work and thereby gain the reward of human well-being.

This opportunity is accompanied by a corresponding threat and a corresponding risk. The threat is that if the child doesn't undertake the work prerequisite to flourishing, it will suffer harm. And we can now see that it will be harmed quite literally, because without the capacities needed for human flourishing, the child will find itself in a position of passive subjection to its circumstances, lacking the resources to cope with them. The corresponding risk is that even if the child accepts the challenge of flourishing, it may nevertheless fail. (The streets of every large U.S. city are littered with individuals who are not coping with their circumstances, or are coping only poorly, and who are consequently faring poorly.)

The opportunity wrapped up in the gift of life is thus an offer of the sort that the child cannot refuse. To be born as a human being is to be handed a job of work, with a promise of great rewards for success, a threat of great harm for refusal, and a risk of similar harm for failure. The scene on which a human child appears willy-nilly is the scene of a predicament, a challenge with very high stakes. Hence the so-called gift of life is indeed a mixed blessing, as Shiffrin claims.

Shiffrin and other philosophers tend to view parental obligations as arising from the harms and benefits that parents confer on children by bringing them into existence. As I argued in the previous part, however, parents are metaphysically incapable of conferring either harms or benefits in that way. The Aristotelian spin that I have now put on Shiffrin's arguments enables me to conceive of parental obligations in different terms.

What is equivocal about procreation is not that it confers both benefits and harms on the resulting child; what's equivocal is that it throws that child into a predicament, confronts it with a challenge in which the stakes are high, both for good and for ill. Moreover, it is a challenge that no child can meet without the daily assistance of others over the course of many years, since the human infant is not at all equipped to acquire the necessary capacities on its own. In my view, those who create a child thereby incur an inalienable obligation to provide the necessary assistance.

Consider the hackneyed example of a child who is drowning at the deep end of a swimming pool. People lounging around the pool obviously have an obligation to rescue the child. But the obligation to fish the child out doesn't fall on the bystanders equally if one of them pushed the child in. The one responsible for the child's predicament is not just a bystander like the others, and he bears the principal obligation.

Obviously, if the responsible party cannot or will not help the child, then others are obligated to act. The child has a right to be saved by somebody if not by the person who caused its predicament. But just as obviously, the person who pushed the child into the pool should have considered beforehand, not just whether someone or other would come to its assistance, but whether he himself was willing and able to fulfill the obligation of assistance that he was about to incur. You shouldn't go pushing children into the deep end if you aren't willing to get wet.

Likewise with procreation and parenting. In my view, parents who throw a child into the predicament of human life have an obligation to lend the assistance it needs to cope with that predicament, by helping it to acquire the capacities whose exercise will enable it to flourish and whose lack would cause it to suffer. By choosing to create a child, perhaps even by choosing to have sex, adults take the chance of incurring this obligation. To risk incurring the obligation without intending to fulfill it is irresponsible; actually to incur it and then not to fulfill it is immoral.

I will shortly consider whether it is morally permissible for biological parents to delegate this obligation to others. Is the obligation incurred through the act of procreation an obligation to see that the child receives the needed assistance in coping with the human predicament? Or is it an obligation to render that assistance oneself, in person?[32]

---

32 Jeff Sebo has directed me to Henry Sidgwick's remarks on the subject: "This ... we might partly classify under ... duties arising out of special needs: for no doubt children are naturally objects of compassion, on account of their helplessness, to others besides their parents. On the latter they have a claim of a different kind, springing from the universally recognized duty of not causing pain or any harm to other human beings, directly or indirectly, except in the way of deserved punishment: for the parent, being the cause of the child's existing in a helpless condition, would be indirectly the cause of the suffering and death that would result to it if neglected. Still this does not seem an adequate explanation of parental duty, as recognised by Common Sense. For we commonly blame a parent who leaves his children entirely to the care of others, even if he makes ample provision for their being nourished and trained up to the time at which they can support themselves by their own labour. We think that he owes them affection (as far as this can be said to be a duty) and the tender and watchful care that naturally springs from affection: and, if he can afford it, somewhat more than the necessary minimum of food, clothing, and education" (*The Methods of Ethics* [Indianapolis: Hackett Publishing, 1981], p. 249).

Of course, parental obligations must sometimes be transferable in practice. A child has a right to grow up in the care of parents who are willing and able to care for it. If its biological parents do not rise to the task, then the child has a right to adoptive parents who are willing and able to take their place. Thus, the mere unwillingness of biological parents to discharge their obligations may be sufficient to ensure that those obligations may be transferred to others, in deference to the rights of the child.

But this practical accommodation does not mean that the biological parents are morally permitted to abdicate their responsibilities at will. We do not think that parents are permitted to relinquish a newborn for adoption because of a last-minute social engagement, for example, or dismay at the size of its ears.

More importantly, we don't think that adults are permitted to conceive a child with the prior intention to put it up for adoption. A woman may not decide to conceive simply in order to have the experience or health benefits of pregnancy, we think, no matter how confident she may be of finding suitable adoptive parents to take over her subsequent responsibilities. Thus, we regard parental obligations as transferable, morally speaking, only under exigencies that make their transfer beneficial for the child rather than convenient for the parents.

In one case, however, we tolerate a practice equivalent to creating a child for adoption. Those who "donate" their sperm and eggs play their role in conceiving children whom they have no intention of parenting. Indeed, they play their role in conception precisely on the condition that they will never be called upon to deal with the resulting children, a condition readily accepted by those who purchase their gametes, which would be unacceptable if they came with parental strings attached.[33] Why do we condone the antecedent intention to transfer parental obligations in this case?

Before I discuss the transferability of parental obligations, I want to discuss a different question raised by donor conception, about the provision that one must be able to make for future children in order to be justified in creating them. People should not create children for whom they cannot provide adequately; but what is an adequate provision? In particular, does

---

33 My discussion of donor conception will be confined to the typical case of anonymous donation between strangers. Cases of donation within families, or of "open" donation, are significantly different in respects that would call for different treatment.

an adequate provision require an opportunity for the child to know and be reared by its biological parents?

Here I am using the word 'adequate' in a sense that is relativized to a particular decision, namely, the decision whether to create a child. Most adoptive parents make more than adequate provision for their adopted children, but the relevant standard of adequacy is premised on the children's already existing and needing a home. My question is what provision for a child is adequate to justify the decision to create it in the first place. And my view is that the standard of adequacy applicable to the procreative decision is different from the standard applicable to decisions made after the child already exists.

My arguments in Part I imply that the adequacy of a child's initial provision is not relative to what could have been provided to the selfsame child. The child will not be in a position to identify his interests with those of the better- or worse-provisioned children he might have been. From the child's perspective, the better or worse starts he could have had in life will not be a matter of self-interest, because his self-concern will extend only to his actual present and possible future selves, not to children inhabiting possible histories that will already have diverged from reality. When the child compares the hand he has been dealt at birth with those he might have been dealt, he will not be able to see himself as ahead or behind in the game of life; he will only see himself as starting a life that amounts to a whole new game. Hence, what could have been provided to him in particular is not especially relevant to the standard of an adequate provision.

A standard that philosophers sometimes apply to procreative decisions is whether the resulting child would have "a life worth living". In Part III of this series, I will argue that this phrase has no meaning that can apply to procreative decisions. 'A life worth living' can mean "a life worth continuing", but procreative decisions concern whether a life should be started, not whether to continue it. Alternatively, 'a life worth living' can mean "a life not to be regretted", but I will argue that people are biased against regretting their existence by considerations that depend on their already existing, considerations that are irrelevant to the decision whether to bring them into existence. In any case, what's barely preferable to nonexistence is not enough for a child by the standard of adequacy that I consider appropriate.

The standard that I consider appropriate does not peg a child's initial provision at any particular level of happiness or well-being. Hence, it is not what philosophers call a person-affecting standard; it is rather a personhood-respecting standard.[34] An adequate initial provision for a child, in my view, is one that expresses due consideration for the importance of human life.

When creating human life, we are obligated to show due consideration for *it*, not just for its individual possessors. The importance of human life itself forbids us to treat it lightly in creating it.

Human life is important because it is a predicament faced by a creature that matters — that is, by a person, whose success at facing it will entail the flowering of personhood, and whose failure will entail a disfigurement of that value, in the form of damage to the self. Just as we are obligated to realize the value of personhood in ourselves, so we are obligated, in creating human lives, to create ones in which that value is most likely to flower and least likely to be disfigured. In this respect, the importance of human life is like the importance of art — the kind of importance that makes something worth creating well if worth creating at all.

Due consideration for the importance of human life requires us to ensure that the human race does not go extinct, but it does not require us to create any particular human lives, or any particular number of them. With respect to individual lives, it mainly requires that we avoid creating lives that will already be truncated or damaged in ways that seriously affect the prospects for personhood to be fully realized within them.

I claim that a life estranged from its ancestry is already truncated in this way. This claim is no less than universal common sense — though it is also no more, I readily admit. I cannot derive it from moral principles; I can at best offer some reflections on why we should trust rather than override common sense in this instance.

When I say that my claim is universal common sense, I mean that people everywhere and always have based their social relationships, in the first instance, on relations of kinship, of which the basic building block is the relation between parent and child. Not every society has favored the nuclear family, of course, but virtually every society has reared children among their kin and in the knowledge of who their biological parents are. The universal consensus on this matter is enshrined in the United Nations

---

34 For a similar view, see Rahul Kumar, "Who Can Be Wronged?", *Philosophy & Public Affairs* 31 (2003): 99-118.

Convention on the Rights of the Child. Article 7, paragraph 1, states: "The child shall be registered immediately after birth and shall have the right from birth to a name, the right to acquire a nationality and, as far as possible, the right to know and be cared for by his or her parents."[35]

When people deny the importance of biological ties, I wonder how they can read world literature with any comprehension. How do they make any sense of Telemachus, who goes in search of a father he cannot remember? What do they think is the dramatic engine of the Oedipus story? When the adoptive grandson of Pharaoh says, "I have been a stranger in a strange land," what do they think he means? How can they even understand the colloquy between Darth Vader and Luke Skywalker? Surely, the revelation "I am your father" should strike them as a piece of dramatic stupidity — a remark to be answered, "So what?"

As the stories of Telemachus, Oedipus, Moses, and even Luke Skywalker illustrate, people unacquainted with their origins have been seen throughout history as dramatically, even tragically, disadvantaged. There must be some reason why people living at different places and times, under very different conditions, have converged on the opinion that a relationship with biological parents is essential to the minimally adequate provision for a child. To be sure, other articles of age-old consensus have been rejected fairly recently in history — the permissibility of slavery, for example. But they have been rejected on the basis of soul-searching reflection, whereas the rise of donor conception has been driven by the procreative preferences of adults, with little thought for the children involved.

Ironically, the preferences of these adults are often based on the same common sense that ought to raise questions on behalf of the children. The reason for resorting to donor conception, after all, is usually the desire of an adult to have a biologically related child despite lacking a partner with whom he or she can conceive. Yet whereas the parent will be just as fully related to the child as any mother or father, the child will know only half of its biological ancestry. These adults seek to enlarge their own circle of consanguinity by creating children who will never know half of theirs. Where is the common sense in that?

As I have said, I cannot prove that knowing and being reared by biological parents is part of the minimally adequate provision for a child; the best I

---

35 For more on the Convention, and some social and legal perspectives on this issue, see footnote 3 in chapter 5 of this volume ("Family History"), and the works cited therein.

can do is to make plausible the venerable and worldwide conviction to that effect. People have tried living in vastly diverse ways, but they have almost always settled on lifeways that accord central importance to biological family ties. Let me offer some considerations that may explain why.

Part of the task facing a human being is to find goals and activities in pursuit of which to develop and exercise the capacities relevant to human flourishing. A human being needs to find work, employment: he needs, as we say, to get a life. A cat does not need to get a life: it instinctively does what it needs to do in order to do well. Getting a life is a task peculiar to the human being, who is not born to do anything in particular, and must therefore figure out what to do with himself.

A human being accomplishes this task by becoming a self worth doing one thing rather than another with. That is, he forms an identity — a complement of traits and attitudes, reflected in a self-image by which to guide their expression in practice. The task of identity formation is not optional for a human being. As soon as he acquires the cognitive wherewithal to ask "Who am I?" and "What am I like?", he is obliged to start coming up with answers, in order to form a specific identity for which there will be specific ways of flourishing.[36]

The task of forming an identity is carried out on raw materials that are not infinitely plastic. A human being begins life with a somewhat determinate temperament and set of aptitudes, which can be kneaded into many different shapes but not into just any shape whatsoever. These individual raw materials are present at birth, as determined by the child's genetic endowment (and perhaps by the intrauterine environment as well).

Research on twins and adoptees has shown that many psychological characteristics are heritable to a considerable degree. Genetic differences are responsible for a proportion of the variance between people not only in IQ (somewhere above fifty percent) but also for the variance in their traits of personality such as extraversion, conscientiousness, agreeableness, and openness to experience (around fifty percent); in whether their interests are artistic, social, enterprising, or conventional (around thirty percent); in their inclination toward authoritarian or conservative attitudes (around

---

36 As Sophia Moreau has pointed out to me, there are cultures in which one's identity is largely dictated by social convention. Even within these cultures, however, the individual remains responsible for a significant degree of self-definition. From our cultural distance, the nineteenth-century British housemaid seems to have been stamped with a prefabricated identity; below stairs, however, that housemaid may have been no less self-defined than we are today.

fifty percent); and even in their degree of religiousness (around thirty percent).[37] These measures of heritability are manifested, for example, in greater similarity between identical twins than between fraternal twins, or between biological siblings reared apart than between unrelated children reared together. In many cases, the effects of genetic endowment tend to increase with age, possibly because the influence of guardians wanes. As people approach adulthood, in other words, they come into their genetic inheritance.

Thus, the predicament into which you were born, though generically human in many respects, was also highly individual, because it required you to fashion an identity out of a genetically inherited supply of raw materials. The possibilities and constraints inherent in those materials gradually came to the fore as you grew up and formed your adult identity.

A few people in the world had already coped or were already coping with predicaments similar to yours in its distinctive features — namely, your biological parents and siblings. Not only did each of your parents form an identity out of a genetic endowment half of which was to become half of yours, but also they jointly forged an identity as a couple, by reconciling between themselves the manifestations of what were to become the two halves of your genetic endowment. Or that's what they did if they *were* a couple. For that very reason, however, you stood to benefit from their being a couple; and for similar reasons, you stood to benefit from their rearing you together with your biological siblings, if any.[38]

---

37 My argument does not rest on any particular quantitative measures of heritability. I cite these statistics only for the sake of suggesting a rough order of magnitude to which psychological traits are probably heritable. In considering the statistics, keep in mind that what accounts for variance among individuals does not necessarily account for variance among groups. For example, individual variance in skin color is largely heritable, but the variance between lifeguards and coal miners is almost entirely due to environment.

    The statistics cited here are drawn from Thomas J. Bouchard, Jr., "Genetic Influence on Human Psychological Traits: A Survey", *Current Directions in Psychological Science* 13 (2004): 148-151. On the heritability of values and religious attitudes, see Laura B. Koenig and Thomas J. Bouchard, Jr., "Genetic and Environmental Influences on the Traditional Moral Values Triad — Authoritarianism, Conservatism, and Religiousness — as Assessed by Quantitative Behavior Genetic Methods", in *Where God and Science Meet: How Brain and Evolutionary Studies Alter Our Understanding of Religion, Volume I: Evolution, Genes, and the Religious Brain*, ed. Patrick McNamara (Westport, CT: Praeger, 2006), pp. 31-60.

38 My arguments in Part I imply that the benefit in question consisted, not in a counterfactual life history that would have been preferable, but rather in an improvement that could have been brought about in your actual future prospects. Of course, if your parents conceived you with the intention of transferring their parental obligations to others, then this benefit may have been ruled out before you existed, hence before you had any future

This claim depends on an assumption about heritability that is politically incorrect, I know. We are supposed to believe that every child is born with the capacity to fulfill any arbitrary human aspiration. In private, however, most parents realize that part of their job is to help their child form realistic aspirations, folded into an identity in which it can truly flourish; and they realize that their ability to do so is greatly enhanced by their ability to recognize in the child various traits, inclinations, and aptitudes that they have seen before, either in themselves or in other members of the family.

In the first instance, of course, family resemblance is physical, and family members usually value the physical resemblances among them. There is a temptation to dismiss this attitude as shallow, but I think that it expresses a deep human need. For as human beings, we need to reconcile our identities as persons with our identities as animals.

The structure of human memory is such as to elicit an identification between the self who remembers and the self of the experience retrieved from memory.[39] Locke thought of that identification as constituting personal identity. Even if his metaphysics was shaky, his phenomenology was impeccable: we certainly seem to have existed at whatever times and places we remember experiencing, so that our sense of persisting through time does not depend on re-identifying our bodies on different occasions. Our relation to our bodies can therefore seem to be contingent. We feel embodied in but not identical to our bodies, and so we can imagine, for example, swapping bodies with other people.

To be born in a human body is thus to be susceptible to alienation from it. We are probably the only animals capable of feeling uncomfortable in our own bodies, even hating them — and loving them, too, for that matter. Coming to terms with our bodily selves is thus a part of the human predicament.

A connection to biological parents helps us to cope with this aspect of our predicament. In infancy we learn to love human faces whose features will eventually be blended in the face that emerges in the mirror as we reach adulthood. We grow into a body akin to the bodies from which we came,

---

prospects to be improved. As I explain at the end of this part, however, it would have been wrong of your parents to conceive a child with the intention of refusing to provide the relevant benefit when it became possible to provide it.

39 I discussed this phenomenon in Part I, and I have discussed it before in "Self to Self" and "So It Goes" (chapter 8 of this volume).

while growing into a personality akin to the ones that animate those other bodies. We thus repeatedly have the sense of becoming our own parents, a common form of intergenerational *déjà vu*. Those who do not know their parents can only wonder who they are becoming. Hence they can only wonder, "How did someone like *me* come to be living in a body like *this*?"

Some people say that they have nothing in common with their parents and siblings. I think that they are speaking figuratively; or maybe they are just in denial. Almost all of us look and sound and feel and move and think like the people from whom we came: a genuine sport of nature is very rare. What is more likely is that a person's similarities to his relatives lie in aspects of himself that don't matter to him, or that he dislikes and rejects. Not valuing commonalities is indeed a way of not having anything in common, figuratively speaking; it just isn't a way of literally having nothing in common.

Someone who doesn't value what he has in common with his relatives may think that he need never have known them in order to forge his independent identity. I doubt it. This person is likely to have defined himself as different from his relatives precisely because they exemplified aspects of himself that he would otherwise have been unable to discern clearly enough to disdain. Learning not to be like his relatives has still involved learning from them: if he had never known them, he might well have ended up more like them.

The point is that biological origins needn't be worth embracing in order to be worth knowing. Someone who doesn't know his relatives cannot even turn up his nose at them. The question for him is not "Shall I follow my progenitors?" but "Am I following them?" and to this latter question he can never know the answer. He can have neither the satisfaction of continuing in their footsteps nor that of striking out on his own, because their footsteps have been effaced.

Even if a child never knows its biological parents, they usually remain significant figures in its life, figures to whom the child is likely to develop an attachment. That's why roughly half of adopted children search for their biological families at some point, and it is why the children of donor conception are now starting to search for their families as well.[40] In my view,

---

40 See footnote 2 of "Family History", chapter 5 of this volume.

the tendency to become attached to unknown parents bears on whether parental obligations are transferable, a question to which I now turn.

Why do these children search for absent parents who can no longer rear them and are unlikely to form a significant relationship with them? Having reached adulthood, haven't they finally made these parents redundant? Apparently not, although we can only speculate why. Here are my speculations.

Humans are unlike other creatures in being at risk for feeling unmoored. We have both an egocentric conception of the world and an objective conception of a creature whose conception it is, a creature who is identical with the "I" at the center of that egocentric conception. Seeing the world from within our own point of view and also from without makes us susceptible to a sense of alienation. Unless we can reconcile these two conceptions of ourselves, we may suffer what might be called existential insecurity — an insecure sense of our own concrete reality.

The creature who I am is securely rooted in the objective order. It is rooted in the objective order not only by being located in time and space but also by its location in the web of causality. It didn't just appear out of nowhere: it is the result of causal antecedents that tie it to the rest of spatiotemporal existence. Of course, I am that creature, and so I didn't just appear out of nowhere, either: I came from the same origins. Yet in order to feel that its connections to the rest of reality are mine, I must find a way of translating them into my egocentric perspective — a way of seeing them from my point of view.

The challenge, in other words, is to identify subjectively with the objective reality of the creature who I am, by seeing how that creature's place in reality can possibly be mine. In order to make that identification, I must see how the connections anchoring that creature in the objective order can have, from my personal point of view, the subjective significance of connections.

But of course, the "I" of my egocentric perspective is a person, for whom connections are most real when they are personal connections, consisting in felt attachments. The way to identify subjectively with the creature who I am objectively is to see its place in the objective world as my place in a personal world. Personal attachments to my causal origins, in the form of my biological parents and ancestors, enable me to experience firsthand the objective reality of the creature who I am. If I lack such subjective correlates for the connections anchoring that creature in objective reality, I am existentially insecure, because I am unable to see from my perspective how its place in reality is mine. That's why people who don't know their origins speak of feeling adrift in the cosmos, out of place in the world.

This sense of rootlessness is especially acute in light of elementary knowledge about the realm of living things. That realm is structured by the life-function of self-replication, which locates every living thing in a chain of progenitors and progeny. To be a living thing is to be a link in that chain. Not to experience oneself as located in that chain is to lack a sense of one's membership in the realm of life, which is the locus of one's membership in reality.

Most people feel a need for a connection to that realm. It can be expressed as a need for roots, for a home — for a family. It is manifested in religious creation stories and cosmologies, in the perpetuation of traditions, and in the ceremonies surrounding ancestors and memorials. The same need naturally leads children to seek an attachment to their biological parents. And it is another peculiarity of human beings to be capable of becoming attached even to figures with whom they are not acquainted.

Many animals become attached to members of their family or group, and they appear to experience grief when these attachments are severed. But they become attached only to others with whom they are acquainted and whom they can recognize by sight or sound or smell. Humans, too, become attached to one another by acquaintance, of course; but they have the unique capacity for attachment to others whom they have never met and wouldn't recognize.

Those who study and counsel adoptees believe that they feel the loss of the birth parents they never knew, and that their sense of loss is comparable to that of children who experience parental death or divorce.[41] How can a child experience the loss of parents with whom it has had no relationship to begin with? The answer is that a child is capable of forming attachments to absent figures, provided that they are present to its thoughts as real objects.

Typically, an object is first presented in thought when it is perceived, whereupon a mental file may be opened to store information received from

---

41 See David M. Brodzinsky, "A Stress and Coping Model of Adoption Adjustment", in *The Psychology of Adoption*, ed. David M. Brodzinsky and Marshall D. Schechter (New York: Oxford University Press, 1990), pp. 3-24; and Steven L. Nickman, "Retroactive Loss in Adopted Persons", in *Continuing Bonds: New Understandings of Grief*, ed. Dennis Klass, Phyllis R. Silverman, and Steven L. Nickman (Washington, DC: Taylor & Francis, 1996), pp. 257-272.

it via perception.[42] Such a file is used for thinking about the thing directly, in a way that is not mediated by a description or a concept. One does not merely have an existentially quantified belief to the effect that something satisfies various predicates; one does not merely have various beliefs whose subject-terms pick out the same thing under various descriptions; one has a mental file that stands for the thing and collects predicates descriptive of it, much as the thing itself unifies a bundle of properties.

Though a mental file is typically connected to its object by a channel of perceptual information, it can also stand for an object without such a connection.[43] If a creature can have intentions with respect to its own mental representations, then it can open and maintain a file intended to stand for a single thing. It must somehow pick out what the file is to stand for, but thereafter it can use the file to treat the thing as an immediate object of thought.

Of course, there is no point in opening a mental file for something that probably doesn't exist or cannot be picked out as its intended referent. But no such risks can deter a child from opening mental files for a biological mother or father with whom it is unacquainted. Every child can be certain of having one and only one such mother and father, to whom it can refer as "my mother" and "my father", and for whom it can therefore open files in the assurance of their standing for unique individuals. The child can fill these files with speculations about its parents, and it can become attached to those parents by thinking about them in this distinctively objectual way.

These considerations about the need and the capacity for attachment to biological parents are what lead me to think that parental obligations are nontransferable. The obligations are nontransferable, I think, because they arise in the context of a personal relationship.

Let us consider the daughter of a sperm donor, so that we can rely on pronomial gender to keep the parties straight. If the mother is like other recipients of donated sperm, she may insist that the girl has no use for her biological father, because he is "nobody to her". This statement is demonstrably false. The *daughter* may be nobody to *him*, because he can

---

42 See Robin Jeshion, "Acquaintanceless *De Re* Belief", in *Meaning and Truth: Investigations in Philosophical Semantics*, ed. Joseph Keim Campbell, Michael O'Rourke, and David Shier (New York: Seven Bridges Press, 2002), pp. 53-74. I am grateful to Jeshion for suggesting this way of expressing what was a vague intuition on my part.

43 Again, see Jeshion, "Acquaintanceless *De Re* Belief".

think of her only under the description "my possible children", never knowing whether he is referring to anyone at all. But to her he is a real person, locatable in thought, no matter how elusive he may be in time and space. Like every human child, she knows that with the word 'father', she can reach down a causal chain to address a single other human who is partly responsible for her existence.

In trying to cope with the predicament entailed by her existence, the daughter can want to be helped, not just by some paternal figure or other, but by the particular father who introduced her into that predicament; who links her to humanity, the realm of life, the causal order; who is her prototype and precursor in personal development; and who could give her a hint of how psyche and soma might be reconciled in her case. Out of those needs, the child can establish a mental representation capable of sustaining an emotional attachment to her father, and she can then frame a demand addressed directly to him, whether or not she knows his earthly address. So personal a demand, so obviously justified, deserves to be answered in person.

I know that my view seems grossly unenlightened. What passes for enlightenment today, however, strikes me as the mirror image of the purported enlightenment of the eugenics movement a century ago. Back then, the people who claimed to know better than common sense believed that a person's biological heritage was all-important; today they believe that it is utterly insignificant. Neither belief is true; either belief can lead to a wholesale violation of rights. The rights violated in the present case are the rights of children.

One objection to arguments like mine is that they seem to cast aspersions on donor-conceived children, by implying that they should never have been born. I do not think that my arguments yield that implication in a form that should give offense; in Part III of this series, I explain why. Another objection is that the children of donor conception are likely to waive any claims they may have on their biological parents. I deal with this objection in Part III as well.

A final objection to my arguments is that donor-conceived offspring have received the gift of life, which they wouldn't have received without the help of a sperm or egg donor. But I have argued that life is not a gratuitous benefit but a predicament with which the recipients require a kind of assistance that they will justifiably call on their biological parents to provide.

Note, moreover, that an obligation undertaken in bad faith cannot be excused by the fact that the party to whom it is owed was better off for its having been undertaken. If my promise to assist you with a risky project gives you the necessary confidence to begin it, then I am still obligated to assist you even if, in retrospect, my defaulting on the promise would not cause you to regret having begun. And if I know in advance that I am going to default on my promise, then I cannot justify issuing it on the grounds that it will induce you to begin a project that you will subsequently be glad to have begun, despite my expected default.

In this last example, my behavior is somewhat analogous to that of a sperm donor, only not quite as bad. The sperm donor doesn't induce his offspring voluntarily to enter the predicament of human life, on the grounds that they will be glad to have entered it; and he doesn't just expect to have an all-things-considered reason to default on those obligations. The sperm donor throws his offspring into the human predicament willy-nilly, on the basis of a positive intention to default on the obligations that he thereby undertakes, since he wouldn't have undertaken them, in the first place, if he hadn't planned to default on them. I don't think that he is morally entitled to bank on his children's forgiveness in this way, even if they do eventually forgive him.

III. Love and Nonexistence[44]

The birth of a child can move us to value judgments that seem inconsistent. Consider, for example, a fourteen-year-old girl who decides to have a baby.[45] We think that the birth of a child to a fourteen-year-old mother will be unfortunate, even tragic, and hence that she should not decide to have one. But after the birth, we are loath to say that the child should not have been born. Indeed, we now think that the birth is something to celebrate — once a year, on the child's birthday.

We may be tempted to say that we have simply changed our minds in light of better information. Before the birth, we didn't know how things would turn out and now we know more. But the birth did not bring to light any previously unknown information relevant to our judgments.[46] Or, at least, I mean to restrict my attention to cases in which it didn't. There may be cases

---

44 This part was presented to the graduate student colloquium at New York University (February 2008); at The Fourth Steven Humphrey Excellence in Philosophy Conference at the University of California, Santa Barbara (February 2008), where the commentator was Mark Schroeder; to an ethics conference at Northwestern University (May 2008), where the commentator was Richard Kraut; to a seminar on the ethical significance of emotions at the Centre for the Study of Mind in Nature (Oslo, June 2008); and to the philosophy department of the University of Illinois at Urbana-Champaign. For comments and suggestions, I am grateful to the participants in these events and to Paul Boghossian, Caspar Hare, Robin Jeshion, Nishi Shah, and Sharon Street.

This part bears some similarity to Larry S. Temkin's "Intransitivity and the Mere Addition Paradox", *Philosophy & Public Affairs* 16 (1987): 138-187. Both seek to show that a combination of views about future persons is not as paradoxical as it seems. The difference between the papers is this: Temkin focuses on failures of transitivity among comparative judgments; I address a different problem, in which the value of a general state of affairs appears inconsistent with the values of all possible instances. I am unsure whether the metaethical solution that I propose for the latter problem is called for by the former.

The paper also overlaps in important respects with Caspar Hare's "Voices from Another World: Must We Respect the Interests of People Who Do Not, and Will Never, Exist?", *Ethics* 117 (2007): 498-523. In the last section of that paper, Hare discusses the difference between *de re* and *de dicto* concern for persons, which is more or less the same difference that I discuss here.

Finally, Jeff McMahan discusses many of the same issues in "Preventing the Existence of People with Disabilities", in *Quality of Life and Human Difference: Genetic Testing, Health Care, and Disability*, ed. David Wasserman, Jerome Bickenbach, and Robert Wachbroit (New York: Cambridge University Press, 2005), pp. 142-171. My approach to these issues is similar to McMahan's in some respects and different in others. The closest similarity is to remarks that he makes about "attachments" on pp. 159ff. The greatest difference is that McMahan analyzes cases of this kind as involving changes of evaluative judgment, whereas I analyze them as involving pairs of judgments that seem inconsistent only if understood in mistakenly realist terms.

45 This case is discussed by Derek Parfit in *Reasons and Persons*, chapter 16.

46 McMahan makes the same point, on p. 155.

in which we feared specific calamities, such as a birth defect or a descent into juvenile delinquency; and then if such possibilities don't materialize, we change our minds. I am not speaking of such cases; I am speaking of cases in which we disapproved of the girl's decision for reasons that are not falsified by subsequent developments and yet we are subsequently glad about the birth. The child is raised under serious disadvantages of the very sort that we anticipated, but the severely disadvantaged child is still a child to be cherished.

We knew in advance how we would feel. Even as we deplored the girl's decision, we knew that we would welcome the child. We may even have cited this prospect to ourselves as a reason for softening our opinion: "Don't condemn her for deciding to have a child," we might have said, "Once it is born, you'll be delighted." But such arguments could not dispel our sense that something was wrong.

One might think that these judgments can be reconciled, after all, because their objects are not the same. When we think that the girl should not have a baby, the object of our judgment is a quantified proposition, about her having some baby or other, whereas it is the birth of a particular baby that we will celebrate.[47] And of course we can consistently think that her having *a* baby is unfortunate in general but not in the case of her having some particular one, since the general rule affirmed by our first judgment may allow for an exception noted by the second.

Yet the attempted reconciliation appears to be blocked by the fact, which was known to us in advance, that any baby she had would be welcomed. How can we judge that a fourteen-year-old's having a baby would be unfortunate as a rule if we also judge that any particular instance of the rule would be an exception?

I do not think that we actually change our minds after the birth of this child, if a change of mind would entail giving up our antecedent judgment. We still think that the girl should not have had a baby, delighted though we are with the baby she has had. That one judgment predominated beforehand and the other afterward should not be allowed to obscure the fact that we are of two minds about the case.

One might hope to dispel the appearance of inconsistency by claiming that the former is a prima facie judgment, deploring any birth only insofar

---

47 This reconciliation is the one that I propose in "Family History", chapter 5 of this volume. I now regard it as inadequate.

as the mother was underage and thus leaving open the possibility of mitigating circumstances. But we don't just think that the girl should not have had a baby insofar as she is underage; we think that she should not have had a baby all things considered; and yet we are glad about the birth of this baby all things considered as well.

The mother herself may regret her decision. She may wish that she hadn't had a baby, may believe that she shouldn't have had one. But of course she still loves the baby and is thankful that it was born. As in our case, her judgments persist in light of one another. That is, she regrets having had a baby when she did even though it was this baby; and she is thankful for this baby even though she had it when she did.

This conundrum is one of several that Derek Parfit considers in Part IV of *Reasons and Persons*, the part devoted to "Future Generations". I want to suggest a solution that Parfit doesn't consider. Parfit's entire discussion presupposes that our value judgments must be consistent as descriptions of the things they evaluate: they must be satisfiable by some distribution of positive and negative value across the possibilities. I think that the present case gives us reason to reject this assumption.

How could it be rational to have such different attitudes toward one and the same event? The answer lies in the different modes of presentation under which the event is viewed.

Our unfavorable judgment is about the baby under a description. What makes this judgment tenable despite our countervailing judgment is not, as we initially suspected, that it is general rather than singular. We think not only that the girl should not have had *a* baby at fourteen but that she should not have had *the* baby she had at fourteen, thus considered under a definite description that picks it out uniquely. The reason why these judgments withstand our favorable judgment about the baby is that, whereas they rely on descriptions, the favorable judgment is about the baby considered demonstratively, as "this baby", "him", or "her".

Why does it matter whether we can make judgments about the baby considered demonstratively? The reason is that such judgments are guided by emotions that depend on acquaintance-based thought. One such emotion is love.[48] In the context of its mother's love, the child is presented to her mind as it is known to her directly via sight and touch. She does

---

48 On the role of perception in love, see my "Love as a Moral Emotion", *Ethics* 109 (1999): 338-374, reprinted in *Self to Self*, pp. 70-109, and "Beyond Price", chapter 4 of this volume.

not love it under descriptions of the form "such-and-such a child" or "the so-and-so" or even as "Fred" or "Sue". The latter modes of presentation would have been available to her even if she had merely heard the child described or referred to by name, in which case she would be in no position to love it. Unlike those modes of presentation, acquaintance-based thought is a way of being mentally in touch or en rapport with an object; and the rapport it entails is prerequisite to the emotion of love.[49]

Our mental relation to something can determine which attitudes toward it are rational. Before we are acquainted with a baby, we can approve or disapprove of it, but loving it is quite impossible, in my view, and hence not rational, either; whereas loving a baby after being acquainted with it is the easiest thing in the world; rational, too.

The different responses that are rational to have toward the baby, as we think of it under different modes of presentation, account for our different value judgments about its birth. We should feel free to experience these responses and hold the corresponding judgments, because value is the shadow of such attitudes, not an independent standard of their correctness. If the attitudes make sense, then the fact that they cast conflicting shadows cannot undermine their authority. And they make sense, despite the conflict between their shadows, because their intentional objects are different in ways that rationally affect the emotions informing our judgments.[50]

---

49 Thus, an expectant mother who says that she already loves her future child may not be speaking the truth, in philosophical strictness. She may be imagining how she will love the child, mentally simulating what it will be like to love the child, or having fantasies of loving it. But until she becomes acquainted with it, her emotion cannot be love.

When does a prospective mother become acquainted with her child? I would say that she becomes acquainted with it when she first perceives it. And when does she first perceive her child? I would say that she perceives the child at the point traditionally called quickening, when the fetus begins to make movements that she can feel. Thus, the tradition that interpreted quickening to be a morally relevant threshold was not just a superstition, in my view; it drew what may indeed be a morally relevant distinction.

50 This dissolution of the problem would be unnecessary if our emotions led us to judgments positing distinct and incomparable values. If we judged merely that the girl's initial decision was imprudent, whereas the baby is beautiful, then we could interpret our judgments as descriptions satisfiable in the one and only actual world, on the grounds that beauty has nothing to do with prudence. Pluralism about values could thus spare us from resorting to antirealism.

But I am imagining us as drawing — as I think we do draw — all-things-considered conclusions about whether a baby, or this baby, should have been brought into existence. And I am imagining that, whereas we still think that the girl shouldn't have had the baby she did, we think otherwise about this baby's having been had. Pluralism about value won't render these judgments compatible.

Parfit considers other ways of dealing with the conflict, but none strikes me as satisfactory. For example, Parfit claims that, were he the child of a birth that was

The child may see his mother's regret, and as he approaches adulthood, he may find the words for what he sees: "You wish you hadn't had a baby when you were so young, don't you?" If the mother is wise enough to realize that she cannot hide her feelings, her answer will be "Yes." "So you wish that I hadn't been born?" No, not at all.

What does the child's second question mean? He is asking whether his mother loves him and is thankful that he exists. But what he wants to hear, in wanting to hear that she loves and cherishes him, is that she loves and cherishes him as the child of her acquaintance, the child she sees and hears and held as a baby in her arms. He doesn't care how she feels about the child she had when she was fourteen, under that description. Let her regret having had the child so described, so long as he himself, as he is known to her directly, can still be sure of her love.

The child may be similarly ambivalent about his own birth considered under different modes of presentation. If he has grown up disadvantaged by his mother's immaturity, as I have imagined, he may conclude from his own experience that the child born to his mother when she was fourteen should not have been born. And yet he may have a healthy self-love that makes him thankful for having been born.

I think that similarly conflicted reactions can arise in the parents of children who are born severely disabled. These parents are, so to speak, doomed to love a child such as is regrettable to have or to be — regrettable, that is, when considered as such a child, not, of course, as this child. In this respect, the parents are caught in a bind partly created by their love for their own child, a bind of a sort that makes the birth of such a child all the more tragic. Similarly, a child born into unfortunate circumstances is doomed to be attached to a particular existence such as is regrettable to have. As an adult, he may resent the fact that his inevitable self-attachment forces him to be thankful for having been given a life of such an unfortunate kind.

Obviously, all-things-considered judgments had better not conflict if they are to provide practical guidance. Before conceiving her child or carrying

---

unfortunate when viewed prospectively, he would agree in retrospect that he shouldn't have been born. I think that he might indeed hold this judgment, but I think that he would also be glad to have been born, so that the former judgment doesn't settle the issue.

    I also prefer this solution to the one favored by McMahan, according to which we change our minds about the girl's decision to have a baby. McMahan considers a solution like mine, when discussing the evaluative import of "attachments to particulars", but he ultimately drops the solution in favor of one based on a change of mind.

it beyond the point where abortion became unavailable, the girl had to choose one way or the other, and we may have been called upon to advise her. Under those circumstances, being of two minds would have been problematic.

Under those circumstances, however, grounds for ambivalence were lacking. Before the child existed, he was not available to be loved or valued in other acquaintance-based ways. The mother's potential love for her child, or his potential self-love, were not antecedent grounds for choosing to create him, since she could not choose to create *him* in particular, considered demonstratively, as he would subsequently be loved.[51] Her choice was not whether to create him but whether to create a child. And of course she should have waited to create a child until she was better prepared to care for it.

Our conflicting value judgments are rationally tolerable because they are retrospective and hence not action-guiding.[52] Given that there is no longer any occasion to make a decision, we can afford to hold conflicting judgments about the decision that was made. The pragmatic drawbacks of ambivalence have fallen away, and the only remaining drawback would be a need to make judgments that reflect some real distribution of value among the former options. In my view, however, there is no such distribution of values, and so ambivalence about the case can be perfectly rational.

My view leads me to question a term that figures prominently in Parfit's work and the literature that it has spawned. The term is 'a life worth living'. I believe that there is no coherent concept attached to this term.

Ordinarily, when we ask whether a life is worth living, we are asking whether it is worth continuing. Then our question is whether the benefits of continuing to live will adequately repay the subject for the associated burdens. An apparent problem with even this ordinary sense of the term is that it requires a comparison where comparison seems impossible. For

---

51 See Matthew Hanser, "Harming Future People", *Philosophy & Public Affairs* 19 (1990): 47-70, p. 61.

52 I do not accept Allan Gibbard's conception of value judgments as hypothetical plans for what to do if in the relevant agent's circumstances (*Thinking How to Live* [Cambridge, MA: Harvard University Press, 2003]). Plans are not evaluative, and evaluations are not plans. When the girl decided to have a baby, the natural expression of her plan would have been "I'm going to have a baby" — not "Having a baby is the thing for me to do." And if she had said, "Having a baby is the thing for me to do," a natural rejoinder would have been "So are you going to have one?" — which would have been an inquiry as to her plan.

whether the benefits of continued life are worth the burdens must depend on the alternatives: any balance of benefits to burdens may in principle be worthwhile if all of the alternatives would be worse. But in the case of continued existence, there is no balance of benefits and burdens with which to compare, since the alternative is nonexistence, in which there would be no subject to whom benefits or burdens could accrue. How, then, do we tell whether life is worth continuing?[53]

This problem is easily solved. When we ask whether a life is worth continuing, we are asking whether the subject has good reason to go on, and such a reason would consist in some event whose inclusion in his life would make it better as a whole. When someone wants to live long enough to finish an important project or have some meaningful experience, he probably thinks that doing so would help to complete his life or bring it closer to perfection.[54] And in that case, he is making a comparison for which the requisite alternatives are to hand — namely, his life extended to include the valued event, on the one hand, and his life cut short without including it, on the other. He can consider whether the one life would be a better life to have lived than the other. If the answer is yes, then he will say that the prospect of the event gives him a reason to live.

But this sort of reason for him to live is not necessarily a reason to be glad that he was born. Having started an important project, he may judge that he will have lived a much better life if he finishes it than if he dies leaving it unfinished; and yet he need not think that his finishing the project will justify his very existence, since the value of finishing the project may be contingent on his having started it. If he had never existed to start the project, his not existing to finish it might have been neither here nor there.

Of course, a life may qualify as not worth living at all if it is not worth continuing from the very outset, in the sense that every increment to its duration makes it a worse life on the whole. But the opposite of being not worth living at all in this sense cannot serve as a standard for which lives are worth living, if that standard is to guide procreative decisions. For we can hardly justify initiating a life on the mere grounds that there would

---

53 Some think that a life is definitely not worth continuing if the benefits of each additional moment are less than the burdens. I do not believe that the value of continuing a life can be reduced to a balance of these momentary values. See my "Well-Being and Time", chapter 7 of this volume.

54 See Bernard Williams's discussion of "categorical desires" in "The Makropulos Case: Reflections on the Tedium of Immortality", in *Problems of the Self: Philosophical Papers 1956–1972* (Cambridge: Cambridge University Press, 1973), pp. 82-100.

not immediately be reason to terminate it. Thus, which lives are worth continuing cannot tell us which lives are worth creating.

Unfortunately, Parfit uses the term 'a life worth living' in the latter sense, and this sense of the term gestures toward a truly impossible comparison. A person cannot compare the value that his life has for him to the value that nonexistence would have had, since nothing has value for the nonexistent.

Parfit offers a solution to this problem. His solution is to ask whether the person, if born, would live to regret it. According to Parfit, the subject's retrospective preference, actual or ideal, between his existing and his never having existed determines whether his life is worth living.[55]

But as I have pointed out, the child of a fourteen-year-old mother may regret the birth of the child his mother had at fourteen while being thankful that he was born. He thus regrets his birth under one mode of presentation but not under another. The question is which attitude determines whether his life is worth living, according to Parfit. My sense is that Parfit wants to give the benefit of the doubt to lives whose subjects would be thus conflicted. That is, he judges a life to be worth living unless the person living it would regret his own birth even when thinking of himself demonstratively. The result is that Parfit takes sides with the inevitable attachment that a person feels for himself by acquaintance — the very attachment that may force him to be thankful for an existence that he thinks undesirable for anyone to have.

My own inclination is to see this preference as rather cruel. I am inclined to say that we should not bring people into lives that they can be thought of as forced to be thankful for. In any case, we cannot assume that there is a fact of the matter as to which criterion of regret we should apply when judging whether lives are worth living. Hence we still lack a determinate comparison that would give a clear meaning to the term 'a life worth living'.

---

55 See p. 487: "[A person] might ... decide that he was glad about or regretted what lay behind him. He might decide that, at some point in the past, if he had known what lay before him, he would or would not have wanted to live the rest of his life. He might thus conclude that these parts of his life were better or worse than nothing. If such claims can apply to parts of a life, they can apply, I believe, to whole lives." In my view, Parfit here misinterprets the comparison that is made by someone who regrets having continued to live after some point in the past. According to Parfit, the person is judging his life since that point to have been "worse than nothing" — worse, that is, than nonexistence. I would say that the person is judging his life with its recent continuation to be worse than the life he would have had without it.

My explanation of our value judgments also bears on the problem that dominates Part IV of Parfit's book, the so-called non-identity problem. In the case of the fourteen-year-old girl, the non-identity problem is supposed to be this: If she postpones motherhood until she is older, she will not have the same child. So the child she has at fourteen cannot be harmed by being born to an underage mother, since *he* cannot be born to a mother who is mature. How, then, can his mother's decision be wrong?

Parfit fleetingly considers what I believe to be the correct solution to this problem. The solution is that a child has a right to be born into good enough circumstances, and being born to a fourteen-year-old mother isn't good enough.

This solution relies on an understanding of rights as including more than morally protected interests.[56] As I argued in Part I, a child's initial provision in life makes no difference to his interests, because he cannot identify his interests with those of the children he would have been if differently provisioned. In Part II, I considered the standard of adequacy for a child's initial provision, arguing that the appropriate standard reflects our obligation to show due consideration for the importance of human life itself. Human life is best seen as a predicament, and the creature thrown into that predicament is a creature that matters, because of being a person, whose success or failure at coping with the predicament will entail the flourishing or withering of personhood.

In creating human lives, then, we must take care that they afford the best opportunity for personhood to flourish. We are obligated to give our children the best start that we can give to children, whichever children we have; and so we are obligated to have those children to whom we can give the best start. A child to whom we give a lesser initial provision will have been wronged by our lack of due concern for human life in creating him — our lack of concern for human life itself, albeit in his case.

If the fourteen-year-old girl decides to have a child, he will probably grow up to be glad that he was born, but he may also feel that he was not given due consideration at his conception. What will have been slighted, from his perspective, is not his well-being but rather the importance of humanity in him — in him, that is, as the instance of humanity that ended up being involved, not as the antecedent target of the slight. For a person

---

56 For this point, and its application to the non-identity problem, see Rahul Kumar, "Who Can Be Wronged?".

can be wronged by being the one who ends up at the receiving end of disregard for the value of humanity in general.

A person suffers such a wrong, for example, when he meets the fate that others risked imposing, not on him in particular, but on someone or other, say, when they chose to dispense with expensive provisions for public safety. And he suffers that wrong even if his interests are not adversely affected — say, because he happens to be nearing the end of a terminal illness. Personhood has been disrespected, and he turns out to be the instance of personhood involved. Such is the wrong suffered by a child who ends up at the receiving end of a mother's disregard for the personhood of her unspecifiable future children.

The child may therefore blame his mother, despite being glad to exist. And whereas his reason for blaming her was available to her antecedently as a reason against having a child, his reason for being glad to exist was not available to her as a reason in favor of having one, since it consists in an attachment that depends on his existence. Hence no considerations of identity or non-identity should have confused the girl about whether to have a child.

Parfit initially seems to think that the right to have been created with due consideration for humanity is a right whose violation can always be excused, on the grounds that the holder of this right wouldn't exist if it hadn't already been violated. Parfit then realizes that it may be wrong to create someone holding an already violated right.

Yet Parfit dismisses this solution to the non-identity problem on the grounds that the child, being glad that it was born, is likely to "waive" its birthright. Since the violated right created by the mother is bound to be waived, he thinks, she is off the hook. Here Parfit's reasoning is confused in two respects, one of which involves the nature of acquaintance-based value judgment. (I'll discuss the other confusion in a footnote.)[57]

---

57 Ordinarily, the prospect of waiving a right arises in the context of three possible outcomes. We can (1) retain the right in order to ensure either (a) that it will be fulfilled or (b) that we will have legitimate grounds to protest its nonfulfillment; or we can (2) waive the right. Entertaining all three outcomes, we may prefer to retain the right, even though we would prefer to waive it if outcome (1)(a) were excluded. That is, we may think that retaining the right for the sake of possibly having it fulfilled would be sensible, but that retaining it merely for the sake of having grounds for protest would be petty and foolish.

Given our preferences, the party against whom we hold the right can induce us to waive it if he can manage to take outcome (1)(a) off the table. But surely a waiver obtained by such means would not be normatively valid. He cannot gain release from

The fact that a child would be glad to have been born does not entail that he would excuse his mother from her procreative obligations. He can reasonably say to his mother, "I'm glad that *I* was born, but you were wrong to have a child in my case." Not only can he reasonably say this; he probably *will* say it, once he realizes that other children have been given, and sensibly regard themselves as entitled to, the best start in life that their parents could provide to a child. He will continue to assert his birthright, despite being glad that he was born.

My attempt to vindicate these seemingly inconsistent judgments depends on the claim that they are based on a rational pair of attitudes. Yet the attitudes themselves may seem irrational precisely because they support conflicting judgments about one and the same event. How can it be rational for a person to be glad, all things considered, about his mother's having done something that he regards, all things considered, as regrettable?

Let me outline a conception of value that supports this claim.[58] I'll start with the relation between value and evaluative response.

There are people whom I like despite knowing that they aren't very likeable, and then there are people whom I know to be likeable even though I just don't like them. Similarly, there are some jokes that I laugh at while judging that they aren't funny, and other jokes in which I can see the humor without being at all disposed to laugh. But when I say that I *find* someone likeable, or *find* something funny, I am doing some third thing. On the one hand, I am not just liking or laughing; I am discovering — "finding" — some quality that merits a response. On the other hand, I am not simply judging that the relevant quality is present; I am finding it with the relevant sensibility, precisely by responding. I am detecting likeability or humorousness with the appropriate detector, namely, liking or laughter.

---

fulfilling our right by confronting us with the fact that he isn't going to fulfill it, so that our only alternative to waiving the right is to retain it for the petty purpose of lodging a protest.

   To be sure, the child of a fourteen-year-old mother cannot exactly claim that she has taken outcome (1)(a) off the table: it was never on the table for this particular child. And yet the child may still waive his birthright because his only alternative is to complain that it cannot be fulfilled. And such a waiver is granted less voluntarily, because it is granted in the presence of fewer relevant alternatives, than the waiver of a right that can still be fulfilled. Its validity is therefore questionable.

58 This conception of value is defended at greater length in my "A Theory of Value", *Ethics* 118 (2008): 410-436, and in Lecture 2 of *How We Get Along* (Cambridge: Cambridge University Press, 2009).

To find someone likeable or admirable or enviable, to find something interesting or amusing or disgusting — these are what might be called *guided responses*, responses that are somehow sensitive to indications of their own appropriateness. Guided responses are not value judgments or evaluations, since they are still conative or affective rather than cognitive. But they resemble judgments in being regulated for appropriateness, and so they are more than mere responses. Finding someone likeable is more judgmental than merely liking him, but it need not entail passing judgment on his likeability. It is rather a matter of liking him in a way that is sensitive to what makes him worth liking. We can mark the partial similarity of such guided responses to value judgments, or evaluations, by describing them as instances of *valuing*.

My analysis of valuing resembles a familiar analysis of action.[59] According to the latter analysis, action differs from mere bodily movement in virtue of being performed for reasons. Bumping into someone, for example, can be an accidental bodily movement, but if one bumps into him for a reason, then it's not just a movement but an action. This analysis of action can be taken as a clue to the nature of reasons for acting. It implies that reasons for acting are considerations such that, when bodily movement is regulated in accordance with them, it rises to the status of action. That is, reasons are considerations whose regulatory influence can make the difference between an accidental collision and a shove.

My analysis of valuing offers a similar clue about reasons for valuing. I have said that finding someone likeable is not just liking him but liking him in a manner sensitive to whatever makes liking him appropriate. But if anything makes liking him appropriate, then it qualifies as a reason for liking him. To find someone likeable is thus to like him for a reason.

---

59 When I speak of action, I mean specifically human action. I agree with Harry Frankfurt that the concept of human action may be "a special case of another concept whose range is much wider", in that it encompasses action on the part of nonhuman organisms ("The Problem of Action", *American Philosophical Quarterly* 15 [1978]: 157-162; reprinted in *The Importance of What We Care About* [Cambridge: Cambridge University Press, 1988], 69-79, p. 79). As Frankfurt explains, the generic concept is that of behavior controlled by the organism, not just one of its constituent subsystems or parts. On this subject, see my "What Happens When Someone Acts?", *Mind* 101 (1992): 461-481; and "Identification and Identity", in *The Contours of Agency: Essays on Themes from Harry Frankfurt*, ed. Sarah Buss and Lee Overton (Cambridge, MA: MIT Press, 2002), pp. 91-128, reprinted in *Self to Self: Selected Essays* (New York: Cambridge University Press, 2005), pp. 330-360. See also my "The Way of the Wanton", in *Practical Identity and Narrative Agency*, ed. Kim Atkins and Catriona MacKenzie (London: Routledge, 2008), pp. 169-192, reprinted in *The Possibility of Practical Reason*, second edition (Ann Arbor, MI: Maize Books, 2015).

What makes for the guided response that amounts to valuing, in other words, is that the response is guided to its target by reasons. And the relevant reasons are those considerations whose guidance would make the difference between merely responding to it and valuing it — between, say, liking someone and finding him likeable, or laughing at something and finding it funny.[60]

If my next step were to say that reasons for liking someone consist precisely in his likeability — that reasons for valuing something, in general, consist in its value — then my analysis would be fairly pointless. No philosophical work would have been done, since value is the term most in need of analysis. My aim is to fill that need, by proposing the opposite order of constitution. Something's value, I want to say, consists in there being reasons for valuing it, which are considerations whose regulatory influence would turn a brute response to it into an instance of valuing. Whatever it is about someone, consideration of which would guide us to like him in a way that amounted not just to liking him but to finding him likeable — *that* is what constitutes likeability. Likeability is that whose detection amounts to finding someone likeable rather than merely liking him; humorousness is that whose detection amounts to finding something humorous rather than merely laughing at it.

The question, then, is how responses are regulated when they are more than casual or haphazard. What is guided laughter or guided liking?

Experimental psychologists have shown that we actually do regulate our responses in accordance with an identifiable set of conditions. We tune our responses so that they make sense in light of our conception of ourselves and our circumstances.

In one experiment, male subjects approached by an attractive female interviewer on a long, wobbly footbridge over a deep canyon showed greater signs of being attracted to her — were more likely to telephone her afterward for a promised debriefing, for example — than subjects approached by the same interviewer on a solid wooden bridge farther upstream.[61] These

---

60 Here I am ignoring the case of acting or responding for bad reasons, which do not actually make the action or response appropriate. The case of bad reasons must be analyzed in terms of good ones, which must therefore be analyzed first.

61 Donald G. Dutton and Arthur P. Aron, "Some Evidence for Heightened Sexual Attraction Under Conditions of High Anxiety", *Journal of Personality and Social Psychology* 30 (1974): 510-517. I review related research in "From Self Psychology to Moral Philosophy", *Philosophical Perspectives* 14 (2000): 349-377, reprinted in *Self to Self*, pp. 224-252. Among

subjects appear to have perceived their anxiety as attraction and acted on that perception. The converse effect has also been demonstrated: subjects are less likely to report or display an emotional response if they have been given an alternative explanation for its symptoms. For example, shy people placed in a socially awkward situation do not feel or act shy if told that they have been exposed to a stimulant that tends to cause the heart to pound.[62]

How does this mechanism work? Attribution theorists generally explain it in terms of a drive toward self-understanding — or, as they prefer to say, toward "cognitive consistency". This cognitive drive gives us a strong incentive to react in ways that we can explain in light of the circumstances, and to behave in ways that we can explain in light of our reaction. Feeling stirred, we look to our circumstances to suggest an interpretation, and we then behave accordingly. In doing so, we can shape an inchoate disturbance into a specific response, or transform one response into another.

Initially we may feel excitations that could be symptomatic, say, of nervousness, fear, or awe. Which of these responses we interpret ourselves as having depends on which response would make sense to us under the circumstances; how we go on to behave depends on how it would make sense for us to behave, given the response we interpret ourselves as having; and we thereby give our initially ambiguous feelings the stamp of nervousness, fear, or awe, depending on which would maximize the overall intelligibility of situation, self, and behavior.

Why do our excitations come to fulfill our interpretation of them? The reason is that our actions feed back into their psychological sources both causally and conceptually. Fearful actions can turn our response into fear partly by shaping the response itself, in the way that smiling has been shown to affect our mood.[63] Fearful actions can also help to constitute which response we are having, since part of what makes the difference between nervousness and fear is how it is manifested in behavior.

---

my claims in that paper is that various disagreements among researchers in this field — which I am glossing over here — are based on misunderstandings that obscure broad areas of agreement.

62 Susan E. Brodt and Philip G. Zimbardo, "Modifying Shyness-Related Social Behavior Through Symptom Misattribution", *Journal of Personality and Social Psychology* 41 (1981): 437-449.

63 See James D. Laird, "The Real Role of Facial Response in the Experience of Emotion: A Reply to Tourangeau and Ellsworth, and Others", *Journal of Personality and Social Psychology* 47 (1984): 909-917; and Sandra E. Duclos, James D. Laird, Eric Schneider, Melissa Sexter, Lisa Stern, and Oliver Van Lighten, "Emotion-Specific Effects of Facial Expressions and Postures on Emotional Experience", *Journal of Personality and Social Psychology* 57 (1989): 100-108.

Rather than accept our response as fear, we can even say, "I refuse to be afraid," meaning that we are interpretively marshalling our excitations into awe or nervousness — or perhaps even shyness — by crediting ourselves with one of those attitudes and following suit in our behavior. If we succeed in making the alternative interpretation stick, then we may indeed have implemented a decision as to our response.

Having noted this way of regulating our responses, we need look no further, I suggest, for the kind of regulation that turns our emotional responses into valuations rather than brute reactions.[64] Reacting becomes valuing when it is regulated by the subject's conception of what it would make sense for him to feel. The considerations whose influence turns reaction into valuation are reasons for valuing, and they turn out to be considerations of intelligibility. So the considerations that make something valuable, by providing reasons to value it, are considerations in light of which valuing it makes sense.

Here I may seem to have turned an obvious explanation on its head. The obvious explanation is that conditions make a response intelligible because they make it appropriate, whereas I have said that conditions make a response appropriate because they make it intelligible.[65] I am well aware of reversing this explanatory order. I do so without apology, on the methodological grounds that it assigns to the explanandum that term which is more in need of explanation. We can explain our responses without invoking evaluative notions, whereas we have difficulty explaining the nature of values at all. If the former explanations can help to provide the latter, progress will have been made.

This methodology is especially helpful, I think, in accounting for the subtle shades of objectivity and subjectivity in our guided responses. On the one hand, the conditions of appropriateness for a response appear to depend on the sensibility that is capable of it. What makes something appropriate to admire depends somehow on what an admiring sensibility is attuned

---

64 For an insightful description of this process as it may take place in child development, see Barbara Herman, *Moral Literacy* (Cambridge, MA: Harvard University Press, 2007), pp. 13-18.

65 In "The Authority of Affect", *Philosophy and Phenomenological Research* 63 (2001): 181-214, Mark Johnston argues that the positive or negative affect involved in a desire can render its motivational force intelligible by presenting its object as "appealing" or "repellent". I am not speaking of intelligibility in this sense; I am speaking instead of the psychological-explanatory intelligibility of a response, in light of its role in a person's mental economy.

to, which is what tends to elicit admiration from a sensibility equipped for that response. On the other hand, the conditions of appropriateness for a response cannot be read off the actual responses of the relevant sensibility. What's appropriate to admire isn't merely what admiring subjects actually do admire. So how can what's admirable depend on the responsiveness of an admiring sensibility without collapsing into whatever actually elicits the admiring response?

This problem comes in varying degrees. To begin with, some things just aren't likeable or admirable, and their lack of likeability or admirability seems to be independent of the subject's perspective. But then we allow for individual differences of taste, which entail that what is likeable or admirable for me needn't be so for you. Even these person-relative values seem to transcend the actual responses of the relevant persons, however, since my likes and dislikes can fail to detect what is really likeable from my perspective. Then again, you and I can criticize one another's sensibilities as needing cultivation or refinement, as if there were an objective criterion of good taste. And yet different values appear to differ in their susceptibility to such a criterion, since we allow more leeway for tastes in liking than in admiration.

How can the conditions of appropriateness for a response be objective in some cases and relative to individual sensibilities in others, while also allowing for rational criticism of those sensibilities, and to different degrees for different reactions? The answer, I suggest, is that the fundamental standard of appropriateness for a response is its intelligibility, which is determined partly by the psychological nature of the reaction itself and partly by differences among individual sensibilities, which can themselves be compared and criticized on grounds of intelligibility.

Consider what makes it intelligible to admire someone. Admiration has a distinctive functional role: it disposes one to emulate the admired person, to defer to him, and to approve of his words and actions. In acquiring these dispositions, one may become either more or less intelligible to oneself, depending on one's other attitudes: beliefs with which the person's opinions may harmonize or clash; ideals that he may or may not exemplify; interests that he may or may not share; likes and dislikes of other people whom he may resemble.

If someone falls short of one's own ideals or ambitions, specializes in what strike one as trivialities, espouses what seem like idiocies, reminds one of a hated foe, and resembles no one else whom one admires, then admiring him would make no sense, and in two respects. First, it's hard to explain why one would acquire a disposition to emulate and defer to someone of that kind; and second, acquiring that disposition would make it hard to figure out how it made sense to behave. Would it make sense to emulate the person's failure in the very pursuits at which one otherwise hopes to succeed? Would it make sense to defer to his judgments contradicting one's deepest beliefs? These questions would have no clear and uncomplicated answers, if one really came to admire him. That's why he isn't admirable, whether or not one admires him in fact.

As this example illustrates, the criterion of appropriateness for a response is holistically interdependent with those for other responses, as are the corresponding values. Whether it makes sense to admire someone who excels at a pursuit to which one has hitherto been indifferent may depend on whether it makes sense to begin taking an interest in that pursuit, which may of course depend on whether it makes sense in other respects to admire the person. Similarly, a state of excitation may need to be diagnosed as either fear or awe or nervousness, but it is unlikely to be all three at once. What's frightening may therefore depend on what's awesome or unnerving, and vice versa. That is, what it makes sense to interpret as, and thereby resolve into, awe may depend on what it makes sense to treat as fear or nervousness instead.

Sometimes different responses may be simply incompatible. Fear, anger, ennui, and disgust tend to dampen amusement, and so it can be difficult to understand why we are laughing at things that would ordinarily frighten, offend, bore, or sicken us.[66] We say, "That's not funny," though sometimes we are laughing as we say it; and then we may add, "So why am I laughing?" This rhetorical question confirms that the unfunny is that which we don't understand laughing at. The reason why we don't understand laughing at something is not that it is unfunny; rather, we don't understand laughing at it because it's boring or offensive or disgusting — or utterly unlike the other things that amuse us — and the resulting incongruousness of laughing at it is the reason why we think it isn't funny, despite our laughter.

---

66 I don't mean to deny the possibility of sick and offensive humor. But these forms of humor usually work by testing the limits of the disgusting or offensive; they fall flat as soon as they cause genuine disgust or offense. We laugh partly out of surprise at what we can see or hear without becoming sick or angry; beyond that point, the laughing stops.

Thus, what it makes sense to be amused by depends in part on what it makes sense to be disgusted, bored, or offended by. And each of these latter responses has its own functional profile, determining how it fits into our self-understanding, perhaps in conjunction with yet other responses. What's admirable or desirable may therefore bear indirectly on what's amusing, by way of what is or isn't boring.

These examples illustrate, further, the idiosyncratic nature of responses and the corresponding values. What makes sense for me to admire is not necessarily what makes sense for you to admire, in light of the functional-explanatory connections between admiration and other responses such as belief, desire, love, hate, fear, and awe, in which you and I may also differ. Each of us can thus have sensibilities in light of which things can be valuable for one of us without necessarily being valuable for the other, because valuing them makes sense for one but not for both.

Idiosyncrasy has its limits, however. There are many responses that all of us tend to have by virtue of our common human nature. Such nearly universal responses include an array of physiological appetites; an aversion to pain, separation, and frustration; an inclination toward pleasure, connection, and the fluid exercise of skill; the inborn and automatic fight-or-flight response; an interest in the human face and form; an initial dislike of snakes, spiders, blood, and the dark; and so on. Given the holism of what makes sense in our responses, these fixed points of human nature constrain most if not all of our values. Some things are desirable for any human being, because desiring them will make sense for anyone; other things simply cannot be desirable, because desiring them won't make sense for anyone. That's not to say that everyone desires the former and doesn't desire the latter; rather, it's to say that everyone would make more sense to himself desiring the former and not desiring the latter, given his natural endowment as a member of the species.

The fixed points of human nature place different degrees of constraint on the intelligibility of different responses. Disgust is directly plugged in to the physiological reactions of gagging and retching; desire is regularly sparked by the appetites, but it can also flare up independently, in response to just about anything; there may be nothing that human nature determines us to admire, and yet admiration is deeply embedded in the network of other attitudes; whereas amusement mostly floats free of the network, except for the few connections through which it is inhibited by fear, disgust, anger, and boredom. What makes sense by way of each response is consequently more or less constrained, depending on its degree of natural connectivity.

I believe that the previously noted shades of objectivity and subjectivity can be explained by these considerations — idiosyncratic differences in how it makes sense to respond, commonalities based in our shared nature, the possibility of responding incongruously and of cultivating more intelligible responses. As the intelligibility of a response is more closely tied to our individual characters, the response is susceptible to more specific guidance from a personal standard of appropriateness; as the intelligibility of a response is more closely tied to our common nature, the response is susceptible to more specific guidance from an interpersonal standard; and a standard of appropriateness may itself be improved, as the corresponding sensibility is rendered more intelligible.

A sensibility can become more intelligible, for example, by following recognizable regularities. Practical reasoning therefore favors cultivating appreciative responses to things that belong to general kinds, kinds that are recognizable, if not by explicit description, then at least by family resemblance. Whatever makes it intelligible for me to laugh at a particular joke — thereby making the joke amusing, at least for me — would make it intelligible for me to laugh at any relevantly similar joke, which would therefore qualify as amusing for me, too.[67] Insofar as I can generalize about what kinds of jokes amuse me, or what kinds of people I admire, I can better understand why I am laughing at a particular joke or emulating a particular person.

Practical reason thus encourages me to identify kinds of jokes, recognizable by family resemblance if not by description, that constitute what is amusing for me. It thereby pushes me toward a position that

---

67 On a particular occasion, of course, the relevant similarity may not be an intrinsic quality of the joke itself: what makes it intelligible for me to laugh on this occasion may be that I'm drunk or nervous, which would make it intelligible for me to laugh at just about anything. Yet I am also under rational pressure to identify kinds of jokes that regularly tend to amuse me by themselves, so that I can comprehend my responses to jokes more generally, without reference to the circumstances. And a joke that's amusing for me on this occasion because I'm drunk or nervous may not be intrinsically amusing for me — not "really" amusing, I might say — because it is not the kind of joke that generally makes it intelligible for me to laugh. This notion of what is "really" amusing (or desirable or admirable or whatever) solves a problem raised by Justin D'Arms and Daniel Jacobson in "The Moralistic Fallacy: On the 'Appropriateness' of Emotions", *Philosophy and Phenomenological Research* 61 (2000): 65-90.

appears to confirm the view that being amusing-for-me is a real, descriptive property of things. The reason why amusingness-for-me comes to seem like a real property, however, is that I have cultivated a sense of humor that is regularly responsive to jokes of recognizable kinds, so that I can understand being amused, when I am amused. The same goes for my senses of admiration, inspiration, disgust, and so on: they have been cultivated under rational pressure to be responsive to recognizable kinds of things, which constitute what is admirable, inspiring, or disgusting for me.

Thus, the notion that values are properties distributed consistently among things or states of affairs is actually the reflection of a pattern into which our evaluative responses tend to fall when regulated in accordance with reasons for responding, which are conditions in light of which a response would make sense. The ultimate criterion of appropriateness for an evaluative response is intelligibility, which can be characterized independently of any postulation of values and can therefore be constitutive of values instead.

Although the most intelligible responses are usually those which are consistent across recognizable kinds of things and coherent with our other responses, departures from this pattern can be more intelligible in isolated cases. After all, intelligibility is a holistic matter of overall explanatory coherence, which sometimes requires trade-offs between alternative marginal gains or losses. And because values are constituted by intelligible responses rather than vice versa, we should tolerate cases in which the most intelligible responses cannot be modeled by a consistent distribution of values: they are simply cases in which the normal pattern of intelligibility doesn't hold.

As I have pointed out, conflicting attitudes can undermine intelligibility by making it difficult to identify an intelligible course of action. But in the case of procreative decisions, some of the most significant attitudes are essentially retrospective — such as love for a particular child, which is not available antecedently to guide the decision. It makes no sense to conceive a child out of love for it, an attitude that will not be possible until it exists. After the child exists, both thankfulness and regret may make sense as responses to it under different modes of presentation; and they may make sense all things considered, as parts of a holistically intelligible set of responses.

Consider again the parents of a severely disabled child. These parents may feel that if they truly love their child, as they unquestionably do, then they cannot lament the fact of having had a disabled child, all things considered; and yet they cannot help lamenting what is unquestionably a lamentable fact. The resulting sense of emotional dissonance can wreak additional damage on the child and the family. In my view, however, there is no dissonance between the emotions themselves; the dissonance is between values that the emotions are mistakenly taken to reflect.

The parents should therefore forget about evaluating their child's existence and feel the emotions that clearly make sense for them to feel. What's intelligible in their responses may cast an inconsistent set of shadows on the world, but they are, after all, only shadows.

Let me turn, finally, to the topic with which I started this series: our obligations to future generations. In Part I, I argued that the inheritance we pass on to future generations cannot harm or benefit them, and that our moral relations to them must therefore be conceived in different terms. In Part II, I argued that our moral relations to future people should be conceived in terms of an obligation to take due consideration for the importance of human life, as the context in which personhood is realized or damaged. In this part, I have argued that the gratitude felt by future persons for their existence will be rationally compatible with resentment over their progenitors' lack of due consideration for human life in their case. The supposed gift of life will therefore be no compensation for the wrong we do in disregarding the possibilities for human flourishing or suffering in the future.

7. Well-Being and Time[1]

A person can fare well either over an extended period or at a particular moment. We evaluate how well a person fares over an extended period when we speak of him as having a good day, a good year, or a good life, or when we speak of such a period as going well for him. We evaluate how a person fares at a particular moment when we say that he is doing well just then. We favor different idioms in these two kinds of evaluation: we are more inclined to speak of a person as having a good life than as having a good moment; and, conversely, we are more inclined to use the terms 'welfare' or 'well-being' to express how well things are going for him at a particular moment than to evaluate how well his life goes as a whole. Nevertheless, evaluations of both kinds are judgments of relational value — of what's good for the person or good in relation to his interests — and so they are both judgments of the person's welfare.[2]

1   This chapter originally appeared in *Pacific Philosophical Quarterly* 72 (1991): 48-77 and was reprinted in *The Metaphysics of Death*, ed. John Martin Fischer (Stanford, CA: Stanford University Press, 1993), pp. 329-357. For comments on earlier drafts I am indebted to Elizabeth Anderson, Fred Feldman, Jonathan Lear, Brian Leiter, Peter Railton, Connie Rosati, Michael Slote, and Nicholas White.
2   In this chapter I assume that a person's welfare is defined by his interests, or what's good for him. According to some theories of the good, however, a person can have interests that do not bear on his well-being, since his interests are not all self-regarding, and his well-being depends only on the fulfillment of self-regarding interests. These theories imply that what has value for a person and what improves that person's welfare are not necessarily coextensive. In my view, proponents of such theories should recognize two distinct ways of measuring the relational value attaching to a person's life: first, the extent to which the life fulfills the person's interests, broadly construed; and second, the extent to which the life fulfills the person's self-interest, or welfare interests. Although I ignore this distinction, I believe that it could be introduced into my arguments with only a loss of simplicity. (Thanks to Peter Railton for bringing this point to my attention.)

What is the relation between the welfare value[3] of a temporal period in someone's life and his welfare at individual moments during that period? And what is the relation between the value of a period and that of the shorter periods it comprises? Is a good day just a day during which one is frequently well-off?[4] Is a good week just a week in which the good days outweigh the bad? Is a good life just a string of good years?

The answer to these questions would be yes if well-being were additive. If the welfare value of a time-period in one's life were equivalent to the sum of momentary well-being that one enjoyed during that period, then a good period would indeed be a period during which one was, on balance, well-off, and a good life would be a life composed, on balance, of good periods. But I doubt whether well-being is additive in this way. Of course, I do not mean to rule out the possibility that the amount of momentary welfare accruing to someone during his life and the welfare value of that life might turn out to be the same. I am simply saying that their being the same would ordinarily be an accident, because the welfare value of a life is not in general determined by, and cannot be inferred from, the amount of momentary well-being that the life contains.[5]

Here I am not merely denying that the value of a life can be computed by the addition of values antecedently assigned to its constituent moments. Computing the value of the whole in this manner, by composition, might be impossible only because the values of the parts had to be computed, inversely, by decomposition. If the only way to assess someone's well-being

---

3   Henceforth I shall frequently drop the modifier and speak simply about the value of someone's life. In all cases, however, I shall be referring to the welfare value of the life — that is, how well it goes for the person living it — rather than to its being morally praiseworthy, aesthetically pleasing, or endowed with significance. (See also ns. 8 and 18 below.) I shall also refer to the welfare value of someone's life as his "lifetime well-being".

4   Amartya Sen interprets the phrase 'being well-off' as referring to something other than well-being. "The former," he says, "is really a concept of opulence" ("Well-Being and Freedom", the second lecture in "Well-Being, Agency and Freedom: The Dewey Lectures 1984", *The Journal of Philosophy* 82 [1985]: 169-221, 195 ff.). Without necessarily rejecting Sen's intuitions about the meanings of these terms in ordinary parlance, I shall stipulate, for the purposes of the present paper, that 'being well-off' refers to the state of having well-being.

5   This statement requires one minor qualification. I can imagine a kind of life whose welfare value would be determined by the amount of momentary welfare accruing to its subject. This would be a life with virtually no narrative structure at all — say, the life of someone who is maintained, from birth to death, in a state of semiconsciousness and inactivity. That this particular life would be only as good as the sum of its good and bad moments is perfectly compatible with my claim that a life's value is not in general a function of momentary well-being.

at a particular moment were to compute the fraction of his life's value that was being realized at the time, then the value of the whole would have to be computed first, and couldn't be derived from the values of the parts.[6] In that case, however, well-being might still be additive in the sense that interests me, since the values of the parts and the value of the whole might still be such that the latter had to equal the sum of the former. What I wish to deny is that well-being is additive in even this sense.

My claim thus militates equally against evaluating a whole life by composition and evaluating its parts by decomposition. In my view, just as assigning values to someone's moments of existence and adding them will not necessarily yield the value of his life, so assigning a value to his life and dividing it among his moments of existence will not necessarily yield their values, either.

My strategy will be to criticize these alternative computations in turn. First I shall presuppose a rough understanding of momentary well-being, and I shall argue, on rather intuitive grounds, that the value of a life need not be the sum of the momentary well-being enjoyed within it. Then I shall argue, on more theoretical grounds, against regarding a person's well-being at a particular moment as a currently realized fraction of his life's value. In neither phase of the argument will I presuppose any particular theory of individual well-being; rather, I'll apply what I take to be common-sense notions of faring well, either over one's entire life or within the confines of a particular moment.

Intuitively speaking, the reason why well-being isn't additive is that how a person is faring at a particular moment is a temporally local matter, whereas the welfare value of a period in his life depends on the global features of that period. More specifically, the value of an extended period depends on the overall order or structure of events — on what might be called their narrative or dramatic relations.[7]

---

6 I believe that James Griffin denies additivity in this sense. He initially says, "We can never reach final assessment of ways of life by totting up lots of small, short-term utilities.... It has to take a global form: this way of living, all in all, is better than that" (*Well-Being: Its Meaning, Measurement, and Moral Importance* [Oxford: Clarendon Press, 1986], pp. 34-35). But Griffin then goes on to say that the values of a life's components should be assessed in terms of the components' contributions to the value of the whole, in such a way that "aggregation" is preserved (see esp. p. 36). Thus, Griffin's objection to the "totting-up model", as he calls it, is an objection to computing values by composition rather than decomposition. (See also pp. 88, 104-105, 144-146.)

7 The notion that the value of a life depends on its narrative structure appears in many works, including Alasdair MacIntyre's *After Virtue: A Study in Moral Theory* (Notre Dame,

Consider two different lives that you might live. One life begins in the depths but takes an upward trend: a childhood of deprivation, a troubled youth, struggles and setbacks in early adulthood, followed finally by success and satisfaction in middle age and a peaceful retirement. Another life begins at the heights but slides downhill: a blissful childhood and youth, precocious triumphs and rewards in early adulthood, followed by a midlife strewn with disasters that lead to misery in old age. Surely, we can imagine two such lives as containing equal sums of momentary well-being. Your retirement is as blessed in one life as your childhood is in the other; your nonage is as blighted in one life as your dotage is in the other.

Yet even if we were to map each moment in one life onto a moment of equal well-being in the other, we would not have shown these lives to be equally good. For after the tally of good times and bad times had been rung up, the fact would remain that one life gets progressively better while the other gets progressively worse; one is a story of improvement while the other is a story of deterioration. To most people, I think, the former story would seem like a better life story — not, of course, in the sense that it makes for a better story in the telling or the hearing, but rather in the sense that it is the story of a better life.[8]

Note that I am not committed to the truth of this value judgment in particular. I offer it merely as an intuitively plausible illustration of the possibility that periods containing equal sums of momentary welfare can have different overall welfare values. (The same goes for most of the value judgments offered below.) Even those who don't agree with the present value judgment, or can imagine disagreeing with it, will at least acknowledge that it is a reasonable judgment to entertain; whereas it would be ruled out a priori if well-being were additive.

One who thinks that a life's value is the sum of the momentary well-being enjoyed therein may seek to explain the outcome of this thought experiment as due to subconscious assumptions that violate the experiment's terms.

IN: University of Notre Dame Press, 1984), chapter 15; and Charles Taylor's *Sources of the Self: The Making of the Modern Identity* (Cambridge, MA: Harvard University Press, 1989), 47 ff.

8   Michael Slote has pointed out to me that my view is at risk of being confused with a view sometimes attributed to Nietzsche, to the effect that literary or aesthetic considerations determine the value of a life. (See Alexander Nehamas, *Nietzsche: Life as Literature* [Cambridge, MA: Harvard University Press, 1985].) I am grateful to Brian Leiter for guidance on this subject.

That is, one may claim that a preference between lives stipulated to contain equal amounts of momentary well-being must arise from a silent refusal to grant the stipulation. Those who prefer the uphill climb to the downhill slide, one may say, are simply assuming that the highs and lows encountered in maturity are more extreme than those encountered in childhood, and that the intensifying effects of age, or mitigating effects of youth, make the goods of one life better and the evils of the other life worse.

But I doubt whether our preference between these lives can be traced to a denial of their supposed symmetry. We don't necessarily assume that the best retirement is better than the best childhood, or that the miseries of age are worse, at their worst, than the miseries of youth. If asked why we prefer the life of improvement, we would be unlikely to express such views; we would be more likely to say, "A life that gets better is, other things being equal, better than a life that gets worse."[9] We would then be expressing a preference between trends, as opposed to sums, of momentary well-being, a preference that is entirely natural and yet at odds with the view that a life's value is the sum of the values of its constituent moments.

This preference can be further sustained by reflection on the counterintuitive consequences of the opposing view.[10] If the value of a life

---

9 Our preferences among trends in well-being are not confined to that for improvement over deterioration. I think that one may have reason to prefer variety and intensity to consistency and moderation — that is, a life of great joys and sorrows to one of uninterrupted contentment — even if the sum of momentary well-being were the same in both lives; or there may be reasons supporting the opposite preference. (Amartya Sen favors equality of well-being among the different moments in one's life. See "Utilitarianism and Welfarism", *The Journal of Philosophy* 76 (1979): 487 f.) As I have said, my argument doesn't depend on showing one such preference to be more rational than another. I am arguing against a view that would deny the possibility of reasons supporting either preference, given the equal amounts of momentary well-being accumulated in the two lives.

10 The point made in this paragraph is borrowed from Connie S. Rosati, who makes it in a somewhat different context. See her "Mortality, Agency, and Regret," *Poznan Studies in the Philosophy of the Sciences and the Humanities* 94 (2007): 231-259. Rosati has pointed out to me that people sometimes regret having started too late on a particular career or relationship, as if the value of their lives has been permanently reduced by this delay in their success or happiness. But I am not committed to denying that there can ever be a bad start that permanently depresses the value of one's life. I am committed only to denying that early misfortunes necessarily depress the value of one's life, as they necessarily would if well-being were additive. What's more, I suspect that the view of well-being as additive cannot properly account for the cases that Rosati has in mind. What these people regret is not the level of well-being that they enjoyed in youth but rather their delay in embarking on a particular project that (as they now realize) will provide an important theme or plot for their life's story. Hence their regret can be understood only as an attitude toward the narrative structure of their lives.

were additive, then a life could be forever spoiled or saved by its initial segment. Every year of well-being would raise the minimum value to which one's life could possibly fall; every year of suffering would lower the maximum value to which one's life could possibly rise. An unfortunate childhood would therefore make for a bad start in life, not only by leaving one emotionally or physically ill-equipped for future challenges, but also by permanently lowering the level of lifetime well-being to which one could reasonably aspire. Conversely, a fortunate childhood would provide not only the personal resources with which to succeed in the future but also so much lifetime well-being in the bank, so to speak, insuring the value of one's life against subsequent reverses. But surely we do not think, after reading the first few chapters of a biography, that they have placed limits on how well or how badly the subject's life might possibly turn out. We don't think, "He's already fifteen years to the good," or "… fifteen years in the hole," as if registering credits or debits that will necessarily be reflected in the subject's final accounts. Yet we do think that we know how well the person fared during the first fifteen years of his life.

My remarks thus far may differ only slightly from, and add only slightly to, what Michael Slote has said in his essay "Goods and Lives".[11] There Slote offers an example closely resembling the cases I have discussed:[12]

> A given man may achieve political power and, once in power, do things of great value, after having been in the political wilderness throughout his earlier career. He may later die while still "in harness" and fully possessed of his powers, at a decent old age. By contrast, another man may have a meteoric success in youth, attaining the same office as the first man and also achieving much good, but then lose power, while still young, never to regain

---

11 In *Goods and Virtues* (Oxford: Clarendon Press, 1983); originally published in *Pacific Philosophical Quarterly* 63 (1982): 311-326. Recently the additivity of well-being has also been challenged by John Bigelow, John Campbell, and Robert Pargetter in "Death and Well-Being", *Pacific Philosophical Quarterly* 71 (1990): 119. Nicholas White has pointed out to me that an early argument against the additivity of well-being appears in C. I. Lewis's *An Analysis of Knowledge and Valuation* (La Salle, IL: Open Court Publishing Company, 1946), chapter XVI. In reading Lewis, I have difficulty separating (1) the claim that the juxtaposition of events in a life affects the value of the whole; (2) the claim that it affects the intrinsic character of the events themselves, which are colored by the recollection and anticipation of other events; and (3) the claim that the value of a life depends on its character as a diachronic experience that is not reducible to a succession of momentary experiences. My defense of (1) does not depend on claims like (2) or (3). My argument can thus be viewed as a generalization of Lewis's, in which I abstract from Lewis's experiential conception of value.

12 In *Goods and Virtues*, pp. 23-24.

it. Without hearing anything more, I think our natural, immediate reaction to these examples would be that the first man was the more fortunate....

Slote goes on to say that our natural reaction to such a case "seems to suggest a time preference for goods that come late in life".

Whether Slote is describing the phenomenon that I have in mind depends on how this last remark is to be interpreted. On the one hand, a preference for goods that come late in life may reflect the view that one and the same commodity, as measured in purely descriptive terms, often adds more to one's well-being if it is received later. In that case, however, the preference in question is perfectly compatible with the view that a life's value is the sum of the momentary well-being enjoyed therein. For even if a particular quantity of pleasure or money or fame gives a greater boost to one's momentary welfare if it is received later in life, what the commodity adds to one's total momentary welfare, whenever it is received, may still exhaust its contribution to the value of one's life overall. On the other hand, the goods among which Slote's temporal preference discriminates might be equilibrated as goods rather than as commodities — that is, in terms of their impact on one's welfare at the time of their receipt. In that case, the preference reflects the view I am defending, that one and the same increment in one's momentary well-being may have greater or lesser effect on the value of one's life, depending on when and how it occurs. Although Slote sometimes appears to favor the former view,[13] only the latter would place him in disagreement with Sidgwick's principle that "a smaller present good is not to be preferred to a greater future good"[14] — a principle with which Slote claims to disagree. I shall therefore interpret Slote's "pure time preference" as implying that a life's value is not equivalent to a sum of momentary well-being.

I hope to build on Slote's observations in two ways. First, I would like to suggest a deeper explanation than Slote's for the preferences cited in his article. While I agree with Slote that two benefits of equal momentary value may contribute differently to the welfare value of one's life, I doubt whether they can do so merely because of their timing. They can do so, I think, because they can belong to different life stories, which coincidentally place them at different times.

---

13 E.g., when saying that "a good may itself be greater for coming late rather than early in life" (ibid., p. 25).

14 *The Methods of Ethics* (Indianapolis: Hackett Publishing Co., 1981), p. 381.

Second, I hope to draw out the consequences of this phenomenon for various issues in moral psychology and moral philosophy. Among the issues I shall discuss are the evil of death, the nature of prudence, and the value of desire-satisfaction.

Consider the theoretical conclusion that Slote hopes to illustrate with the case cited above:[15]

> When a personal benefit or good occurs, [it] may make a difference to how fortunate someone is (has been), quite independently of the effects of such timing in producing other good things and of the greater importance we attach to the distinctive goals and interests of certain life periods. And I believe, in particular, that what happens late in life is naturally and automatically invested with greater significance and weight in determining the goodness of lives.

While I agree with Slote's evaluative intuitions about the case, I do not agree with this explanation of them. The reason why later benefits are thought to have a greater impact on the value of one's life is not that greater weight is attached to what comes later. Rather, it is that later events are thought to alter the meaning of earlier events, thereby altering their contribution to the value of one's life.

Suppose that we drew one of Slote's politicians behind a veil of ignorance about his life and put to him the following proposition. He is to have ten years of political success, but he can choose whether his fortunate decade is to occur in his fifties or his thirties. How strong a preference would he have between the alternatives thus described? I suspect that he would be indifferent.[16] If he had any preference at all, it would be neither

---

15 Michael Slote, *Goods and Virtues*, p. 23.

16 Here I am assuming that the veil of ignorance deprives the subject of information about his current age. For if he knew that he was currently in his forties, then he might have a preference arising out of what Derek Parfit calls the bias toward the future (*Reasons and Persons* [Oxford: Oxford University Press, 1984], 165 ff.). Note, then, that the time preferences considered by Slote are different in structure from those considered by Parfit. Parfit is concerned with a preference between past and future, whereas Slote is concerned with a preference between early and late. As the subject's temporal relation to an event changes, the former preference yields a different attitude toward the event, but the latter does not. Connie Rosati has suggested to me that a person might prefer earlier success because it would be a sign of genius. But this suggestion strikes me as only proving my point. The person so described would not prefer earlier success merely by virtue of its timing; he would prefer it only because he values the meaning of some story that its early occurrence would subserve.

as strong nor as stable as the preference he would have if we described the alternative careers more fully, as they are described in Slote's example. Merely postponing a fixed amount of well-being until later in life wouldn't strike him as an obvious means of making it more valuable; indeed, he might reasonably regard well-being as more valuable if enjoyed in youth. Surely, then, the preference elicited by Slote's example must depend on something other than the effects of mere timing.[17]

In order to reproduce the preference elicited by Slote's example, we would have to tell the aspiring politician that the later successes being offered to him would be the culmination of a slow ascent, whereas the earlier successes would be the prelude to a sudden decline. That is, we would have to tell him, not only about the timing of the rewards in question, but also about their place in a larger trend. He wouldn't care whether a particular bundle of goods was to be encountered early or late in the game; what he would care about is whether they were to be encountered at the top of a chute or the top of a ladder.

Why would a person care about the placement of momentary goods on the curve that maps his changing welfare? The answer, I believe, is that an event's place in the story of one's life lends it a meaning that isn't entirely determined by its impact on one's well-being at the time. A particular electoral victory, providing a particular boost to one's current welfare, can mean either that one's early frustrations were finally over or that one's subsequent failures were not yet foreshadowed, that one enjoyed either fleeting good luck or lasting success — all depending on its placement in the trend of one's well-being. And the event's meaning is what determines its contribution to the value of one's life.[18]

---

17 Bigelow, Campbell, and Pargetter also express doubts about Slote's treatment of this case. See "'Death and Well-Being'", pp. 122-123.

18 To say that the meaning of an event determines its contribution to the value of one's life is not to equate a valuable life with a meaningful one. To be sure, meaningfulness is a valuable characteristic in a life, and it, too, is probably a function of the life's narrative structure. But we can conceive of meaningful lives that aren't particularly good ones for the people who live them; and we may be able to conceive of good lives that aren't particularly meaningful. What's more, the meaning, or narrative role, that determines an event's contribution to a life's value, in my view, must not be confused with the event's meaningfulness in the evaluative sense. To say that a particular increment in momentary well-being adds more to the value of a particular life if it has the meaning of a well-earned reward than that of a windfall is not to say that rewards are necessarily more meaningful events; it's simply to say that their contribution to the life's value depends on their being rewards.

The meaning attached to a quantity of momentary well-being is determined only in part by its place in the overall trend.[19] The meaning of a benefit depends not only on whether it follows or precedes hardships but also on the specific narrative relation between the goods and evils involved. Slote's politician would have experienced an improvement in his well-being whether his years of toil were capped by electoral victory or merely cut short by his winning the lottery and retiring young. But the contribution of these alternative benefits to the overall value of his life wouldn't be determined entirely by how well-off each would make him from one moment to the next. Their contribution to his life's value would also be determined by the fact that the former would be a well-earned reward, and would prove his struggles to have been a good investment, whereas the latter would be a windfall in relation to which his struggles were superfluous. Thus benefits that would effect equal improvements in his momentary well-being might contribute differently to the value of his life, by virtue of lending and borrowing different meanings in exchange with preceding events.

The most familiar illustration of this principle is the commonly held belief in the importance of drawing lessons from one's misfortunes. If a life's value were a sum of momentary well-being, learning from a misfortune would be no more important than learning from other sources, since every lesson learned would add so much value and no more to the sum of one's well-being. On being invited to learn from a personal tragedy, one would therefore be entitled to reply, "No, I think I'll read a book instead." Edification would offset the losses incurred in the tragedy, but its having been derived from the tragedy wouldn't render edification more valuable, either intrinsically or extrinsically. Any lesson of equal value would offset one's losses equally.[20]

---

19 Here I disagree with Bigelow, Campbell, and Pargetter, who believe that the value of someone's life, though not reducible to the sum of the momentary well-being enjoyed throughout that life, nevertheless supervenes on the pattern of the person's momentary well-being through time. (See "Death and Well-Being", pp. 127-128, 136-137.) Indeed, these authors believe that momentary well-being just is that property — whatever it may be — whose profile through time determines the value of a person's life (ibid., p. 128). My reasons for rejecting this view are expounded in greater detail below.

20 In some cases, of course, what we hope to learn from a misfortune is how to avoid repeating some mistake that occasioned it. But why do we think it more important to learn how to avoid repeating a past mistake than to learn a different lesson, about how to avoid committing a novel mistake? The reason isn't that we regard the consequences

The point of learning from a misfortune, surely, is to prevent the misfortune from being a total loss. Learning from the misfortune confers some value on it, by making it the means to one's edification. But how could this be the point? The instrumental value of a means is not to be counted as additional to the intrinsic value of the end. Otherwise, we would be obliged to pursue our ends as circuitously as possible, so as to accumulate the most instrumental value along the way. Since the value of a means is not additional to that of the end, turning a misfortune into a means of learning a lesson doesn't produce any more value than that inherent in the lesson itself, a value not necessarily greater than that of any alternative lesson one might have learned. So how can the point of learning from a misfortune, in particular, be to confer instrumental value on it?

The answer, I believe, is that conferring instrumental value on a misfortune alters its meaning, its significance in the story of one's life. The misfortune still detracted from one's well-being at the time, but it no longer mars one's life story as it formerly did. A life in which one suffers a misfortune and then learns from it may find one equally well-off, at each moment, as a life in which one suffers a misfortune and then reads the encyclopedia. But the costs of the misfortune are merely offset when the value of the latter life is computed; whereas they are somehow cancelled entirely from the accounts of the former. Or rather, neither misfortune affects the value of one's life just by adding costs and benefits to a cumulative

---

of a repeated mistake as necessarily worse than those of a mistake committed for the first time. We might prefer committing a novel mistake to repeating a past mistake even if their consequences would be equally bad. Surely, the reason is that we regard the story of committing the same mistake repeatedly as worse than that of committing different mistakes — a value judgment that depends on more than the momentary costs of the mistakes themselves. One might think that our interest in learning from misfortunes, and the mistakes that occasion them, is based on the assumption that the mistakes a person has already committed are the ones that he's most likely to commit in the future, and hence that lessons learned from them are the ones that are most likely to be useful. I disagree. We value learning from mistakes even if we know that the opportunity to repeat them will never arise. And we value learning from misfortunes, such as grave illnesses or freak accidents, that are not in any way attributable to mistakes. Finally, one might think that learning from a misfortune is valuable only because it is a means to a more pleasant consciousness of the misfortune — a means of "coming to terms" or "making peace" with it. But why not simply forget about the misfortune entirely, or turn one's thoughts to something else? If making peace with a misfortune were valuable only as a means to pleasurable consciousness, then any alternative pleasure would serve just as well. Making peace with a misfortune is valuable not just because it entails acquiring so much peace of mind but because it entails acquiring peace of mind in a way that draws a fitting conclusion to one's past. (All of the objections considered in this note were suggested to me by Connie Rosati.)

account. The effect of either misfortune on one's life is proportionate, not to its impact on one's continuing welfare, but to its import for the story. An edifying misfortune is not just offset but redeemed, by being given a meaningful place in one's progress through life.[21]

The same point can be illustrated with other examples. In one life your first ten years of marriage are troubled and end in divorce, but you immediately remarry happily; in another life the troubled years of your first marriage lead to eventual happiness as the relationship matures. Both lives contain ten years of marital strife followed by contentment; but let us suppose that in the former, you regard your first ten years of marriage as a dead loss, whereas in the latter you regard them as the foundation of your happiness.[22] The bad times are just as bad in both lives, but in one they are cast off and in the other they are redeemed. Surely, these two decades can affect the value of your life differently, even if you are equally well-off at each moment of their duration. From the perspective of your second marriage, you may reasonably think that your life would have gone better if you could have made your first marriage work out; and you may reasonably think so without thinking that the first marriage, if successful, would have been better from day to day than the second. You can simply think that a dead-end relationship blots the story of one's life in a way that marital problems don't if they lead to eventual happiness.

Of course, your desire for a successful first marriage is fulfilled in the latter life, whereas in the former it is given up and replaced by the desire for a successful second marriage. In a sense, then, the former life differs from the latter by virtue of containing more unfulfilled desires. Doesn't this

---

21 Charles Taylor remarks on our concern for whether the past "is just 'temps perdu' in the double sense intended in the title of Proust's celebrated work, that is, time which is both wasted and irretrievably lost, beyond recall, in which we pass as if we had never been" (*Sources of the Self*, p. 43). Taylor goes on to say that our desire to prevent the present from becoming lost in this sense is a desire for "the future to 'redeem' the past, to make it part of a life story which has sense or purpose". Taylor continues: "In the scene in the Guermantes's library, the narrator recovers the full meaning of his past and thus restores the time which was 'lost' in the two senses I mentioned above. The formerly irretrievable past is recovered in its unity with the life yet to live, and all the 'wasted' time now has a meaning, as the time of preparation for the work of the writer who will give shape to this unity" (pp. 50-51).

22 Of course, we can also imagine a life in which an unsuccessful first marriage teaches you lessons instrumental to the success of your second. But in that case, I would claim, your life would be better than it would have been if the first marriage had been a dead loss.

difference in desire fulfillment explain the difference in perceived value between these lives?

I doubt whether a difference in desire fulfillment can do this explanatory job. Suppose, for example, that in both versions of the story your early desire to achieve happiness with your first mate was accompanied by an equally strong, competing desire to start afresh with someone else. The only difference between these desires, let us say, was that during your ten years of trying to fulfill the former, the latter remained an idle yearning on which you never acted. Now the two endings of your story no longer differ in respect to the fulfillment of your youthful desires: each ending fulfills one and frustrates one of the desires that you harbored throughout your first marriage. Do they consequently result in equally valuable lives? I am inclined to say not. For I am still inclined to prefer the ending in which your initial efforts are redeemed over the ending in which they are abandoned. Fulfilling a desire on behalf of which you have struggled may be more important than fulfilling a desire in which you have made no investment. Hence desire fulfillment per se is not what's valuable; what's valuable is living out a story of efforts rewarded rather than efforts wasted.[23]

Insofar as the fulfillment of one's past desires is valuable, I am inclined to say, its value depends on that of life stories in which desires are eventually fulfilled. For I cannot see how a difference in the fulfillment of past desires can yield any difference in momentary well-being. Let us cancel the assumption that you always wanted to change mates, and return to the assumption that the beginning of your story, in either version, includes only a desire to make a go of your first marriage — a desire that's fulfilled in one version but abandoned in the other. The question remains when you are rendered worse off, in the version that involves a second marriage, by the abandonment of your hopes for the first. Once you abandon those hopes, you acquire new ones — for success in the second marriage — and these are richly fulfilled. You are therefore just as well-off in your second marriage, from day to day, as you would have been in your first, had it flourished. To be sure, you are no longer achieving what your former self wanted you to achieve — namely, success in the first marriage — but this

---

23 Peter Railton has pointed out to me that I seem to be appealing to a desire that was omitted from my calculation of desire fulfillment — namely, your desire for a life in which your efforts are rewarded. But I do not think that your desire for a life in which your efforts are rewarded is contingent on the assumption of your having that desire in the life under consideration.

failure can hardly make your former self worse off retroactively. The daily well-being of your former self is a feature of the past, beyond alteration. Failure to fulfill your previous desires thus impinges on your interests without affecting your welfare at any particular moment.

Oddly enough, several philosophers have asserted the possibility of retroactive effects on well-being — often in order to explain when a person suffers the evil of death.[24] According to these philosophers, a person's death can make him worse off during the immediately preceding portion of his life, by preventing the fulfillment of the desires he has during that period.

These philosophers argue that our resistance to the idea of being currently harmed by future events is based on the false assumption that one cannot be harmed by things that don't affect one's conscious experiences. But acknowledging the possibility of unexperienced harms should not necessarily lead us to acknowledge the possibility of present harms due to future events. For even if a person's current welfare is not determined entirely by facts within his experience, it may still be determined entirely by facts within the present.

This restriction on the determinants of momentary well-being cannot be inferred directly from the impossibility of backward causation. Future events could affect one's present well-being if present well-being were a relation between one's present desires and the states of affairs that fulfilled or failed to fulfill them. In that case, retroactively harming someone would no more require retrograde causation than retroactively "making a liar" of him. But momentary well-being is ordinarily conceived as a temporally local matter, determined by a person's current circumstances, whether experienced or unexperienced. We think of a person's current well-being as a fact intrinsic to the present, not as a relation that he currently bears to his future. We don't say, of a person who dies in harness, that he fared progressively worse toward the end, simply because he was acquiring more and more ambitions that would go unfulfilled. Nor do we say, of a person raised in adversity, that his youth wasn't so bad, after all, simply because his youthful hopes were eventually fulfilled later in life.[25] We might say

---

24 These philosophers include Joel Feinberg (*Harm to Others* [New York: Oxford University Press, 1984], 79 ff.) and Bigelow, Campbell, and Pargetter ("Death and Well-Being", pp. 134-135, 138). Note that in rejecting the notion of retroactive effects on a person's momentary well-being, I do not necessarily reject the notion that the value of a person's life can be influenced by events after his death. The reason is that I regard the value of a person's life as a feature of his life story, and a person's life story may not end at his death.

25 Indeed, I don't see how Feinberg or Bigelow et al. can say that such a person's life gets better at all if, in adulthood, he desires that his youth had gone differently.

that such a person's adulthood compensated for an unfortunate youth, but we wouldn't say that it made his youth any better. Because the belief in retroactive welfare effects would entail such judgments, it strikes me as highly counterintuitive.

Thus, the reason why it is generally in your interests to promote the fulfillment of your current desires for the future cannot be that their future fulfillment will make you better off now. Nor can it be that their future fulfillment will make you better off then — that is, better off than you would be if you replaced them with different desires that got fulfilled.[26] The reason why it is in your interests to promote the fulfillment of your current desires for the future is rather that a life story of ambitions conceived, pursued, and fulfilled may be a better life story than one of ambitions conceived, discarded, and replaced. And the one life is better than the other even though they may include equal amounts of momentary well-being.[27]

My view of lifetime well-being provides a different explanation from Slote's for the discrepancy in our attitudes toward early and late stages in life. My explanation begins with the observation that events in a person's life can borrow significance from both preceding and succeeding events. A particular success can be either a windfall or a well-earned reward, depending on the amount of effort that preceded it; the expenditure of a particular effort can be either a good investment or a waste, depending on the degree of success that ensues. Retrospective significance — that which is gained from subsequent events — is often responsible for the discrepancy between total momentary well-being and lifetime value. For when subsequent developments alter the meaning of an event, they can alter its contribution to the value of one's life, but they cannot retroactively change the impact that it had on one's well-being at the time.

---

26 Many philosophers have noted the absence of any rational requirement to satisfy desires that one had in the past (Derek Parfit, *Reasons and Persons*, chapter 8; Richard B. Brandt, "Two Concepts of Utility", in *The Limits of Utilitarianism*, ed. Harlan B. Miller and William H. Williams [Minneapolis: University of Minnesota Press, 1982], p. 180). To my knowledge, these philosophers do not raise the further question of why one has any present reason to promote the fulfillment of one's desires for the future, given that one may have no reason to promote their fulfillment at the time. See also Amartya Sen, "Plural Utility", *Proceedings of the Aristotelian Society* 81 (1980-1981): 202-204.

27 C. I. Lewis offers many suggestive remarks to the effect that striving and achieving have value only as related to each other in a diachronic whole (*Analysis of Knowledge and Valuation*, 498 ff.). As I have noted, however, Lewis's remarks often rely on the notion that the *experiences* of striving and achieving suffuse one another or add up to an irreducible diachronic experience.

From the perspective of practical reasoning, in which the past is fixed but the future remains open, earlier events seem more susceptible to retroactive changes of significance. Even after the events of one's youth have occurred, their import for one's life story remains undetermined, since the events from which they will gain significance or to which they will lend significance lie primarily in the future. By contrast, the events of one's old age occur in the determinate context of one's past, with which they exchange fixed implications that are unlikely to be significantly modified in what remains of one's life. Thus, one looks forward to a lifetime in which to redeem one's youth, but confronts events of middle age as having a single, determinate significance once and for all.

The result is, not that later events are more important, but that one sees less latitude for arranging them within the requirement of a good life. By middle age, one finds oneself composing the climax to a particular story — a story that is now determinate enough to be spoiled. Virtually any beginning might have been the beginning of a good life; but given one's actual beginnings, there may now be only a few good ways of going on.[28]

Because one will confront one's prime with relatively narrow criteria of success, one is required to devote more care to planning it and to ensuring that it turns out as planned. The extraordinary attention paid to this stage in life may be misinterpreted as indicating that it is more important — that the events of middle age contribute more to a life's value than events at other stages. The reason for paying more attention to one's prime, however, is not that the possibilities at middle age are worth more than at other stages but rather that, in relation to a fixed youth, fewer of the possibilities will result in a life that's any good at all.

My account of the value judgments canvassed above amounts to the claim that the value of one's life is what might be called a strongly irreducible second-order good.[29] A second-order good is a valuable state of affairs consisting in some fact about other goods. Of course, corresponding to

---

28 Subsequently, such constraints may relax to some extent, since the events of one's retirement may be less intimately related to the other events in one's life than those occurring at the culmination of one's active career. A life story that has only one fitting climax may have more than one fitting denouement.

29 As Michael Stocker points out, the value of a life is what G. E. Moore would have called an "organic whole" (*Plural and Conflicting Values* [Oxford: Oxford University Press, 1990], pp. 300-302, 323).

every good that someone might attain is the potential fact of his having thereby attained something good; and his having attained something good would undeniably be a good state of affairs consisting in a fact about other goods. There is therefore a second-order good corresponding to every attainable good of the first order. But such a second-order good is reducible to the first-order good implicated in it, in the sense that it has no value over and above that of the implicated first-order good. That is, when someone attains a good, he is not enriched by its value plus some additional value attaching to the fact of his having thereby attained something good. If he were, then he would be infinitely enriched, since the second-order good would generate a good of the third order, and so on ad infinitum.

In order for a second-order good to be irreducible, it must at least possess value over and above that of its component first-order goods. A possible example of such a good in the realm of social value is that of a just distribution of benefits. Some people think that there can be value in redistributing benefits among the members of a society even if the redistribution doesn't increase the total amount of good accruing to individuals. This thought implies that the resulting distribution has a value over and above that of the goods being distributed, and hence that the new distribution is an irreducible second-order good.

There is yet a stronger form of irreducibility that may or may not attach to a second-order good whose value is additional to that of its components. Consider two possible views about the second-order value of a just distribution. On the one hand, we might judge that a distribution of individual benefits has a second-order value that depends entirely on the proportions among the shares of benefits distributed; on the other hand, we might judge that the justice of a distribution, and hence its value, depends on whether individuals deserve their shares by dint of their actions or characters. The first view implies that the value of a just distribution, though additional to that of the benefits distributed, can still be computed from the amounts in which those benefits are distributed. The view thus implies that facts about second-order value are still, in a sense, reducible to facts about mere quantities of first-order goods. By contrast, the second view implies that no facts about quantities of first-order goods can fully determine the facts about second-order value, since the latter also depend on facts about the conduct and characters of individuals. The second view thus implies that the second-order value of a just distribution is irreducible in a stronger sense.

The existence of second-order goods that are irreducible in either sense entails the existence of more than one dimension of value. If social justice is an irreducible second-order good, for example, then there must be a dimension of value other than total individual welfare — a dimension of social value, as it might be called — along which value can be produced even while total individual welfare remains constant.

In the case of distributing benefits among the periods in someone's life, however, the corresponding implication may initially seem odd. If we regard a particular temporal distribution of well-being as having irreducible second-order value for a person, we would seem committed to claiming that its value lies along a dimension distinct from that of total individual well-being, since we shall have said that value can be produced by a redistribution that leaves total well-being constant. Yet the distribution in question is supposed to be good specifically for the person, and so its value would seem to lie along the dimension of individual well-being rather than along any alternative dimension. We are therefore confronted with a puzzle. If a temporal redistribution of benefits produces no additional benefits for the person, how can it be beneficial to him? How can a person be better off under an arrangement that affords him no additional benefits?

The answer to this question is that the value of a temporal distribution of benefits needn't lie along a dimension of value distinct from that of individual well-being; its dimension of value must be distinct only from that of *momentary* individual well-being, since momentary benefits are the benefits whose total remains constant under the envisioned redistribution. Thus, regarding a temporal distribution of benefits as an irreducible second-order good requires the assumption that a person's well-being has both a synchronic and a diachronic dimension. The value of someone's life lies along the dimension of diachronic welfare, which is distinct from, and irreducible to, how well off he is at each moment therein.

Here we find, in a new guise, the value judgment with which I began — namely, that two lives containing equal sums of momentary well-being need not be equally good lives if their momentary benefits stand in different temporal or, more generally, different narrative relations. We can now see what this intuitive judgment implies: it implies that self-interest is not a unitary dimension of value. Rather, a person has two distinct sets of interests, lying along two distinct dimensions — his synchronic interests in being well off at particular moments, and his diachronic interests in having good periods of time and, in particular, a good life.

Although Slote regards a life's value as weakly irreducible, he doesn't regard it as irreducible in the stronger sense.[30] Slote analyzes the values of lives in terms of weights assigned to momentary goods in accordance with the time of their occurrence. He says that some periods of life are more important than others, and hence that the goods and evils occurring in those periods are accorded greater weight when the value of a life is computed. His view therefore amounts to the claim that facts about the value of a life can be reduced to facts about the amounts and temporal order of the momentary benefits enjoyed therein — in short, to facts about temporal patterns of momentary benefits.

In my view, however, the facts about a life's value are not even reducible to this extent. Some of the value judgments considered above are incompatible with any reduction of diachronic well-being to synchronic well-being, no matter how sophisticated an algorithm of discounting and weighting is applied. Because an event's contribution to the value of one's life depends on its narrative relation to other events, a life's value can never be computed by an algorithm applied to bare amounts of momentary well-being, or even to ordered sequences of such amounts, in abstraction from the narrative significance of the events with which they are associated. How the value of one's life is affected by a period of failure combined with a period of success, for example, cannot be computed merely from the timing of these periods and the amounts of well-being they contain. Their impact on the value of one's life depends as well on the narrative relations among the successes and failures involved. Were one's travails in the political wilderness ended by ascent to high office? or were they ended by a lucky ticket in the lottery and a round-the-world cruise? Was one's perseverance through rocky times vindicated or discredited by the particular way in which one eventually attained domestic happiness? Our evaluative intuitions about the importance of learning from misfortunes, or of salvaging one's projects, thus imply that the value of a life is more strongly irreducible than Slote suggests.

---

30 The same goes for Bigelow, Campbell, and Pargetter, who argue that the value of someone's life supervenes on the pattern of his momentary well-being through time. They say, "Surely if two people have had the same temporal well-being at all times of their life-spans of equal length, they are to be seen to have had equal global well-being" ("Death and Well-Being", p. 137). I say: Surely not. For if one person's later good fortune redeemed his earlier sufferings and the other's did not, the value of their lives might well differ.

The degree of irreducibility between second- and first-order goods determines the degree of independence between the corresponding dimensions of value. If we analyze the second-order value attaching to different patterns of benefits in terms of weights attached to those benefits, we shall continue to regard diachronic well-being as reducible to synchronic well-being, albeit by means of a time-weighted algorithm. The implication will therefore remain that the greater weight attached to some goods and evils, because of their occurring at important times, can be offset by a greater amount of goods and evils occurring at times of less importance. The second-order value of a benefit's timing will thus be conceived as exchangeable for a greater amount of that or any other first-order benefit.

Thus, if the problem with a downward trend in well-being were that more importance attached to what happens in one's prime, then there would have to be some amount of childhood happiness that was sufficient to compensate for midlife misfortunes even after the appropriate weights had been applied. Childhood well-being would still amount to so much credit earned toward a good life, even if that credit was computed at a discounted rate. Hence a life that took a slide would still be a good one if it started from a sufficient height.

If we suppose, however, that the second-order value of a life is simply not computable from the amounts and temporal order of the momentary benefits that it contains, then we must conclude that some second-order goods may not be exchangeable for goods of the first order (and vice versa). That is, there may be some undesirable turns of plot whose disvalue simply cannot be offset by greater amounts of momentary well-being in the associated prelude or denouement. I find this implication more consonant with our evaluative intuitions than the implications of Slote's view. It explains why we think that the value of someone's life remains almost entirely undetermined even after he has passed an especially happy or unhappy childhood; and why we are inclined to perceive some wisdom in Solon's refusal to declare Croesus happy without knowing how his life would ultimately turn out.[31]

I therefore favor the principle that a person's self-interest is radically divided, in the sense that he has an interest in features of his life that

---

31 Herodotus, I. 30-33. This story is cited by Aristotle (*Nicomachean Ethics* I.x. 1-2), whose final definition of happiness (at I.x. 15) also betrays an inclination to agree with Solon to some extent.

aren't at all reducible to, and hence cannot be exchanged with, patterns of momentary well-being. Let me briefly suggest two possible applications for this principle.

First, I think that this principle, if correct, justifies a revision in the philosophical conception of prudence and imprudence.[32] Imprudence has traditionally been conceived as an irrational preference for momentary goods that are closer in time, and prudence as a rational indifference toward the timing of such goods. Prudence and imprudence have thus been conceived as dispositions to value momentary goods differently. In my view, however, we should consider the hypothesis that imprudence is rather an undue concern for momentary goods altogether, and prudence, a rational appreciation for the second-order value of a good life — a disposition that cannot be constituted out of any appreciation for patterns of momentary goods. According to this hypothesis, a person can be imprudent no matter how carefully he balances momentary goods of the present against those of the future if he does so without regard to the value of the resulting life, a value not reducible to temporal distributions of momentary goods; and a person can be prudent even if he pursues present benefits at the expense of future benefits, so long as the value of his life is thereby enhanced. Preferring the lesser but nearer good to that which is greater but more remote may sometimes be the prudent thing to do, if done in the service of one's irreducible second-order interest in a good life.

A second application for the principle of divided self-interest has to do with the evil of death. A prevalent view about death is that it is bad for a person if, but only if, his continued survival would add to his accumulation of momentary well-being. The choice between heroic medical treatment and passive euthanasia is therefore frequently said to require so-called quality-of-life considerations. Whether days should be added to or subtracted from a patient's life is to be judged, according to the prevalent view, by whether the days in question would be spent in a state of well-being or hardship.[33]

---

32 Some philosophers seem to regard 'prudence' as synonymous with 'self-interested rationality' or 'practical wisdom'. In this paragraph I am discussing prudence in a narrower sense, in which it denotes a specific aspect of practical wisdom — namely, a rational attitude toward the future.

33 For a clear presentation of this view, see Fred Feldman, "Some Puzzles About the Evil of Death", *The Philosophical Review* 100 (1991): 225-227. Feldman's own view on the matter may not correspond to the view that he presents in this paper, since the paper adopts a simplistically additive hedonism merely for the sake of arguing with Epicureans. What Feldman does believe is that the evil of a particular death must be computed as the difference between the value of the actual life in which it occurs and that of the same

In my view, however, deciding when to die is not (despite the familiar saying) like deciding when to cash in one's chips — not, that is, a decision to be based on the incremental gains and losses that one stands to accumulate by staying in the game. It is rather like deciding when and how to end a story, a decision that cannot be dictated by considerations of momentary well-being. Hence a person may rationally be willing to die even though he can look forward to a few more good weeks or months;[34] and a person may rationally be unwilling to die even though he can look forward only to continued adversity. The rationality of the patient's attitude depends on whether an earlier or later death would make a better ending to his life story.

Thus far I have presupposed a prior understanding of what it is to be well-off at a particular moment, and I have argued that the value of a person's life is not reducible to his momentary well-being, so understood. The reader might be moved to object, however, that I am not entitled to my initial presupposition. One might think that the only legitimate conception of a person's well-being is that of his life's value, and that any conception of his well-being at a particular moment must therefore be illegitimate insofar as it fails to capture the portion of his life's value being realized at that moment.

I shall argue against this suggestion on grounds more theoretical than those of my previous arguments. First I shall offer a more theoretical explanation of why a person's momentary well-being might fail to be additive. The reason, I shall claim, is that a person's well-being at each moment is defined from the perspective of that moment, and values defined from different perspectives cannot necessarily be added together. This explanation will prompt the suggestion that the successive perspectives defining momentary well-being simply distort the true values of things, which are properly defined from the comprehensive perspective of an entire life. I shall then argue against this suggestion, by defending the independent validity of momentary perspectives. Finally, I shall explore some further implications of these theoretical results.

---

life in the nearest possible world in which the death doesn't occur. I do not in general accept this method of computing the value of events in someone's life, since I believe that events have a momentary value that's distinct from their contribution to the value of the subject's life as a whole. Since death has no momentary disvalue, however, my view about it coincides with Feldman's. I discuss this subject further below.

34 Griffin expresses doubts about this view in n. 33, p. 355, of *Well-Being*.

That momentary well-being might not add up should come as no surprise: values are rarely additive. Notoriously, the value of two things together need not be the sum of their individual values.[35] The value of having two egg rolls on one's plate is less than the sum of the values of having one or the other of them; and the value of having one egg roll and a dollop of plum sauce is more than the sum of the values of having either an egg roll or plum sauce alone. To be sure, the value of having two egg rolls is indeed the sum of their marginal values: marginal values are additive. But marginal values are additive only because they are defined by decomposition of total value, to begin with. That is, the marginal value of one's second egg roll is defined as the amount by which its acquisition increases one's total well-being; and this definition guarantees that the acquisition of a second egg roll increases one's well-being by the addition of its marginal value. The point previously made by saying that the values of egg rolls aren't additive can then be made by saying that the marginal values of two successive egg rolls aren't the same.

Of course, what's currently at issue is not additivity in the value of some commodity such as food but additivity in well-being itself. The question is not whether two egg rolls are twice as good as one but whether being well-off at two different times is twice as good as being well-off at one time. And we might have thought that although successive helpings of food can vary in their impact on one's well-being, and hence in their marginal value, successive helpings of well-being cannot.

This thought might have been correct if the helpings in question were defined in relation to the same context of evaluation. But since helpings of momentary well-being are defined in relation to different contexts, they aren't additive at all. Let me explain.

The reason why the marginal value of successive egg rolls varies is that the value of acquiring an egg roll depends on the context in which the acquisition occurs. One's second egg roll is worth less than the first because it is acquired in the context of one's already having the first. Of course, once the second egg roll is assigned a marginal value, that value needn't be further adjusted because of its being acquired in the context of the well-being that's already, so to speak, on one's plate; the egg roll's marginal value already reflects the only adjustment necessitated by the context.

---

35 See Griffin, *Well-Being,* pp. 36, 144-146.

Nevertheless, we often restrict the context in which judgments of value are made. For example, we make distinct assessments of how well-off someone is in different respects — assessments of his financial well-being, say, or his emotional well-being, and so on. And such evaluations are made within restricted contexts. An assessment of someone's financial well-being may take account of the diminishing marginal value of dollars:[36] his second million needn't be thought to make him twice as well-off, financially speaking, as the first. But our assessment of someone's financial well-being does not take account of interactions between his finances and other goods. The impact of a million dollars on someone's overall well-being may depend not only on how much wealth he already has but also on his emotional state or his health. But the potential interactions between wealth and these other goods are screened off from assessments of specifically financial well-being. Two people with equal assets and liabilities (and, perhaps, similar attitudes toward money) are judged to be equally well-off, financially speaking, even if those assets and liabilities affect their overall welfare differently by virtue of their differing emotional or physical circumstances.[37]

Consequently, we cannot compute a person's overall well-being at a particular moment by adding up his concurrent financial well-being, emotional well-being, physical well-being, and so on. The problem is not simply that we don't know how to commensurate among wealth, health, and sanity — that is, how to bring these commodities under a common unit of value for the purposes of addition and subtraction. The problem is that such restricted assessments of well-being are made in isolation from potential interactions among the goods involved. Our assessment of the person's financial well-being doesn't reflect how his emotional and physical circumstances affect the marginal value of his wealth; our assessment of his emotional well-being doesn't reflect how his physical and financial circumstances affect the marginal value of his sanity; and so forth. Thus, even if we could establish an equivalence of value between a

---

36 In speaking of financial well-being, of course, I am assuming that wealth has intrinsic value for a person. Nothing in my argument depends on this assumption. Emotional, social, or physical well-being can be substituted in my arguments, mutatis mutandis, for financial well-being.

37 Assessments of emotional, physical, and professional well-being thus involve what Sen would call "informational constraints" — that is, constraints on which sorts of information are relevant. In Sen's terms, the reason why people with equivalent financial holdings have the same level of financial well-being is that they belong to the same "isoinformation set" as defined by the applicable informational constraint. See "Moral Information", the first lecture in "Well-Being, Agency and Freedom", pp. 169-184.

helping of financial well-being and a helping of physical well-being, we wouldn't have established that the combination of the two was worth twice as much as either one alone, since our measures of financial and physical well-being would not reflect potential interactions between the values of the underlying commodities.

We can easily forget this limitation on evaluative calculations if we imagine value itself to be a commodity. If we picture financial well-being as an elixir distilled from piles of money, we shall think of it as having an independent existence; and we shall then be inclined to think that when financial well-being is added to the values distilled from physical health or emotional stability, the resulting brew must simply be the sum of its ingredients. But an amount of financial well-being is not a quantity of stuff; it is rather a property of one's financial state. Indeed, it's a property that one's financial state possesses only in relation to other possible financial states, just as one's overall well-being at a particular moment is a relation of one's overall state to the other states that one might be in. And there is no reason to assume that the relation of one's overall state to its possible alternatives can be computed from the relations of its parts or aspects to theirs.

The problem of compounding values is analogous, in many respects, to problems in the compounding of chances. Notoriously, the probability of a person's having the trait *p or q* is not necessarily equal to the probability of having *p* plus that of having *q*, since the latter probabilities may not be independent; and for the same reason, the probability of having the trait *p and q* is not necessarily equal to the product of the probabilities of having the component traits. Consequently, we cannot estimate how unusual a person is by compounding the degrees to which he is physically unusual, psychologically unusual, socially unusual, and so on. The product of these probabilities may not reflect the extent to which the person possesses physical and psychological traits that are individually rare but often combined, or vice versa. This computation would therefore count someone with red hair and a hot temper as doubly unusual,[38] even if these two unusual traits tend to go hand in hand; and it would correspondingly underestimate the rarity of someone who is both beautiful and modest. In estimating how physically unusual a person is, we do take account

---

38 For ease of expression, I have chosen to compare probabilities on a logarithmic scale. That is, I call *p* doubly unlikely in relation to *q* if the probability of *p* is equal to the probability of *q* squared.

of interactions among the probabilities of physical traits (red hair and freckles); in estimating how psychologically unusual he is, we take account of interactions among the probabilities of psychological traits (hot temper and romantic passion); but in neither case do we consider interactions between physical and psychological probabilities. Because these estimates of probability are thus confined to different contexts, they cannot be added or multiplied together.

In short, calculating someone's overall well-being by adding up his physical and emotional welfare is no more appropriate than calculating how unusual he is by compounding his physical and emotional quirkiness. My view is that momentary well-being lacks additivity for the same reasons. Estimates of momentary well-being are made within a restricted context — namely, the context of the events and circumstances of the moment. How well-off someone is judged to be at one moment doesn't reflect potential interactions between the value of what obtains and happens then and the value of earlier or later events. Hence evaluations made in the context of one moment cannot be added to evaluations made in the context of another. Being well-off on two occasions doesn't necessarily make a person doubly well-off, any more than being both physically and psychologically unusual makes him doubly unusual.[39]

Again, we shall tend to forget this limitation on evaluative calculations if we imagine an amount of momentary well-being as a quantity of stuff, derived from the facts of the moment but then having an independent existence of its own. In reality, one's well-being at each moment is a relation between the facts of the moment and alternative possibilities; and there is no reason to assume that the relations of successive facts to their alternatives determine the relation of the entire succession to its alternatives.

My claim that momentary well-being is assessed from a restricted perspective might seem to undermine my earlier claim that a person's self-interest is divided. Doesn't my latest argument show that a person's synchronic interests are divided from his diachronic interests only in the sense that his financial interests, say, are divided from his interests as a whole? Either division, one might think, is merely an artifact of the restrictions placed on the context in which synchronic or financial interests are assessed: a person's interests, comprehensively considered, are still unified.

---

39 See the preceding note.

Although I agree that the division between synchronic and diachronic interests results from the difference between the perspectives from which they are assessed, I hesitate to assume that the more comprehensive of these perspectives has exclusive authority. In the case of a person's financial interests, of course, I am inclined to say that insofar as they diverge from his interests overall, they should be regarded as a figment of a restricted perspective and should be ignored. Although a person can limit his attention and concern to financial matters from time to time, the resulting value judgments, even if correct, have no independent authority on which to stand in competition with more comprehensive judgments of his interests.

A person's synchronic interests, however, strike me as having an independent claim that is not necessarily overridden by that of his diachronic interests. The reason, I think, is that a person himself has both a synchronic and a diachronic identity. The perspectives from which synchronic interests are assessed, unlike the financial perspective, are not optional points of view that a person may or may not adopt from time to time. They are perspectives that a person necessarily inhabits as he proceeds through life, perspectives that are partly definitive of who he is. An essential and significant feature of persons is that they are creatures who naturally live their lives from the successive viewpoints of individual moments as well as from a comprehensive, diachronic point of view.

To think that the more comprehensive of these perspectives must have greater authority is, I believe, to mistake how perspectives bear on questions of relational value. When we choose between competing theories about one and the same phenomenon, the more comprehensive theory may be preferable, other things being equal. But the different perspectives currently in play aren't competing theories about the same phenomenon: they're partly constitutive of different phenomena — that is, different modes of relational value. Because well-being is a relational value, it is constituted, in part, by a point of view — namely, the point of view inhabited by the creature whose well-being is in question. What's good for that creature, in particular, depends on what point of view it inhabits by virtue of being the particular creature it is.

Thus, although the perspective of a particular creature is less comprehensive than that of the entire universe, evaluations relative to the creature's perspective aren't any less authoritative than those relative to the universe's point of view. Evaluations relative to a particular creature's perspective are authoritative about what's good for that creature; and what's good for a particular creature is really and truly good for that creature, even if it isn't good for the universe. These two perspectives aren't two competing theories about one and the same mode of value; they're constitutive of two different modes of value.

Similarly, evaluations from the perspective of a single moment in someone's life needn't be less authoritative than those which are relative to the perspective of his life as a whole. Both are judgments of relational value, which is constituted in either case by a particular point of view; and evaluations relative to either point of view are authoritative about what's good from that point of view.

The question, then, is not whether what's good from the perspective of a moment in someone's life is really good, since it really *is* good from that perspective. The question is rather whether the perspective in question has a subject — whether there really is a creature whose perspective it is and who therefore is the subject of the values it constitutes. To this latter question, I think, the answer is yes. By virtue of being who you are, you unavoidably occupy successive momentary viewpoints as well as a diachronic one; and just as what's good from the latter viewpoint is good for you as protagonist of an ongoing life, so what's good from the former viewpoints is good for you as subject of successive moments within that life.[40]

Note that in arguing for the validity of synchronic perspectives, I am not defending or attacking any thesis about time preferences.[41] I am not trying to show that one is entitled to take a greater interest in the present moment than in other moments in one's life. In my view, no one momentary

---

40 This argument is in the same spirit as the following remarks of Thomas Nagel's: "Human beings are subject to ... motivational claims of very different kinds. This is because they are complex creatures who can view the world from many perspectives ... and each perspective presents a different set of claims. Conflict can exist within one of these sets, and it may be hard to resolve. But when conflict occurs between them, the problem is still more difficult. ...[Such conflicts] cannot, in my view, be resolved by subsuming either of the points of view under the other, or both under a third. Nor can we simply abandon any of them. There is no reason why we should. The capacity to view the world simultaneously from [different points of view] is one of the marks of humanity" ("The Fragmentation of Value", in *Mortal Questions* [Cambridge: Cambridge University Press, 1979], p. 134). (Here I have made strategic deletions from Nagel's remarks in a way that may exaggerate their similarity to my view.)

41 I am therefore making a somewhat different point from one made by Bernard Williams. When Williams says, "The correct perspective on one's life is *from now*", he is criticizing the principle that one should "distribute consideration equally over [one's] whole life" ("Persons, Character and Morality", in *The Identities of Persons*, ed. Amélie Oksenberg Rorty [Berkeley, CA: University of California Press, 1976], pp. 206, 209).

perspective takes precedence over any other. My brief is on behalf of all momentary perspectives equally, against the assumption that their deliverances are to be overridden by those of the diachronic perspective that subsumes them. I am trying to show that the value something has for someone in the restricted context of a single moment in his life is a value that genuinely accrues to him as the subject of that moment, even if interactions with events at other times result in its delivering a different value to him in his capacity as the protagonist of an entire life. The good that something does you now is not just the phantom of a restricted method of accounting; it's an autonomous mode of value.

If I am right about the autonomy of synchronic interests, then a person's well-being at a particular moment cannot be computed from the fraction of his life's value being realized at the time, any more than the value of the whole can be computed from the values of its parts. To assess the benefits that someone is currently receiving in terms of their share in the value of his life would be to evaluate everything in the more comprehensive context. Such a method of evaluation might be appropriate for Tralfamadorians, who don't live one moment at a time,[42] but it isn't appropriate for human beings. Just as evaluating a life by adding up the values of its component moments entails neglecting the perspective that encompasses the unity of those moments, so evaluating moments in a life by dividing up the value of the whole entails neglecting the perspectives that preserve their individuality. Each moment in a life is, momentarily, the present. And for a human being, the present is not just an excerpt from a continuing story, any more than the story is just a concatenation of moments.[43]

What if a creature cannot adopt a perspective that encompasses a particular combination of goods? How then do we assess what value the combination has for him or how the values of its components interact?

Consider a nonhuman animal such as a cow or a pig. I assume that a cow cannot conceive of itself as a persisting individual and consequently

---

42 Kurt Vonnegut, Jr., *Slaughterhouse-Five or, The Children's Crusade: A Duty-Dance with Death* (New York: Dell Publishing, 1969), p. 23: "The Tralfamadorians can look at all the different moments just the way we can look at a stretch of the Rocky Mountains. … They can see how permanent all the moments are, and they can look at any moment that interests them. It is just an illusion we have here on Earth that one moment follows another one…."

43 C. I. Lewis also defends the autonomy of momentary value (*Analysis of Knowledge and Valuation*, 503 ff.). Again, Lewis's argument is based on an experiential conception of value.

cannot conceive of itself as enjoying different benefits at different moments during its life. What the cow cannot conceive, it cannot care about; and so a cow cannot care about which sequences of momentary goods it enjoys. The cow cannot care twice as much about faring well at two distinct times than it cares about faring well right now — not because it can care only less than twice as much, but rather because it cannot care at all, being unable to conceive of itself as persisting through a sequence of benefits.

The upshot is that any judgment we make about the value that a particular sequence of benefits has for a cow will bear no relation to how the cow would or should or even could feel about that sequence of benefits. And this result seems incompatible with even a weak form of internalism about value, which would at least rule out the possibility that something can be intrinsically good for a subject if he is constitutionally incapable of caring about it. I am not sympathetic to stronger versions of internalism, which make a thing's intrinsic value for someone contingent on his being disposed to care about it under specified or specifiable conditions; but I am inclined to think that unless a subject has the bare capacity, the equipment, to care about something under some conditions or other, it cannot be intrinsically good for him.[44]

Of course, we can adopt yet a weaker form of internalism, which allows for intrinsic goods that the subject cannot care about, so long as they are compounded out of goods that he can. But this version of internalism will be unstable, for two reasons.

One reason is that this version will commit us to constrain some of our judgments about intrinsic relational value within the bounds of internalism and yet to make other, similar judgments that exceed the same bounds. If we assume that what cannot be of concern to a creature can nevertheless have intrinsic value for that creature provided that it is divisible into components that can be of concern, then we shall need to adopt some method for combining the values of the components. In order to add up the momentary goods enjoyed by a cow, for example, we shall have to make some assumption about how the values of those goods interact, so that we can compute their combined value. And this assumption will constitute another judgment of intrinsic relational value. To suppose that a cow's momentary well-being consists in this or that feature of its current

---

44 Note that internalism applies only to matters of intrinsic value. Obviously, something that's beyond a person's powers of comprehension can still be good for him extrinsically, since it can be conducive to things that are good for him intrinsically.

circumstances is one value judgment; but to suppose that the values of the cow's good moments can be combined in this or that way is a further value judgment, a judgment to the effect that two moments containing the relevant feature are this much or that much better for the cow than one.

Whether we say that one moment of such-and-such a kind is good for a cow, or that two such moments are thus-and-so much better for the cow, we are making a judgment of intrinsic relational value. Yet the proposed version of internalism will say that the validity of the former judgment depends on the cow's ability to care about the object of evaluation, whereas the validity of the latter does not. On what grounds can this distinction be drawn? Surely, whatever intuitive reasons we have for applying the internalist constraint to the first value judgment are likely to be reasons for applying it to the second.

Another, related instability in the resulting view is that it is at odds with a fundamental intuition about relational value — namely, that the value something has for a particular creature is somehow grounded in or determined by that creature's point of view.[45] Insofar as we commit ourselves to combining the values accruing to a subject from goods whose combinations exceed his comprehension, we shall find ourselves making relational value judgments that are not appropriately related to the subject's perspective. There is nothing about the perspective of a cow that supports one assumption rather than another about how the value of two momentary benefits stands to the value of either benefit alone, given that sequences of such benefits are beyond the cow's ken and thus, as it were, nothing to the cow. The combined value would therefore have no claim to represent what's good for the cow, or what's good from the cow's perspective.[46]

---

45 Of course, the intuition expressed here may not be independent of that expressed in internalism. Indeed, there are some interpretations of internalism according to which the two intuitions are one and the same. I separate them here because I regard internalism as resting on a rather different intuition.

46 This point follows most clearly from desire-based conceptions of well-being, which will define how valuable different sequences of harms and benefits are for a cow in terms of how much the cow wants those sequences, or would want them under some ideal conditions. Since a cow cannot care about sequences of harms and benefits, and wouldn't be able to care about them except under conditions that transformed it into something other than a cow, these definitions imply that temporal sequences cannot be assigned a value specifically for a cow. Although my point thus follows from desire-based conceptions of relational value, it does not presuppose that relational value is desire-based. Judgments of relational value must somehow be relativized to the subject's perspective — if not by being made to depend on the subject's actual or counterfactual desires, then by some other means. And any strategy for relativizing evaluations of temporal sequences to the perspective of a cow will run into the same obstacle —

Note that this problem is equally acute for all possible assumptions about how the cow's momentary benefits should be combined. Even the assumption that two equally good moments in the cow's life are twice as valuable as one presupposes a flat curve of marginal value;[47] and this presupposition has no basis in the cow's point of view. Such a straightforward method of adding benefits may have the advantages of simplicity and salience in comparison with other methods, but these advantages shouldn't be mistaken for truth. In respect to truth, any method of combining the values of a cow's good and bad moments will be purely arbitrary and consequently defective, insofar as it fails to represent what values things have specifically for the cow rather than from some other perspective.

I therefore think that we should refuse to combine the momentary benefits and harms accruing to a cow; we should conclude, instead, that a cow can fare well or ill only at particular moments. Good and bad things can befall a cow, but they are good or bad for it only at particular times and thus bear only a time-indexed sort of value. There is no timeless dimension of value along which the cow progresses by undergoing successive benefits and harms. Hence the various benefits accruing to a cow at different moments must not add up to anything at all, not even to zero: they must simply be unavailable for addition.

As before, if we imagine the cow's momentary well-being as a commodity, then we shall be puzzled by the claim that amounts of this commodity cannot be added together. But once we realize that the cow's momentary well-being is a relation that the cow's current state bears to other possible

---

namely, that the perspective of a cow doesn't encompass temporal sequences at all. (One might think that Peter Railton's version of the desire-based conception would have the resources to circumvent this problem, since it would define what's good for the cow in terms of what an idealized cow would want its actual self to desire ["Moral Realism", *The Philosophical Review* 95 (1986): 163]. The idealized cow, one might think, could acquire the ability to conceive of, and form preferences among, temporal sequences of harms and benefits while still doing so on behalf of its cognitively limited and hence fully bovine self. This suggestion strikes me as out of keeping with Railton's theory, for various reasons, of which one will suffice for now: The cognitively enhanced cow, once fully informed, would realize that its actual self was unable to want temporal sequences of harms and benefits, and would therefore not bother wanting its actual self to have any such desires.)

47 See Griffin, *Well-Being*, p. 145: "Even when one does tot up, say, many small-scale pleasures to get an overall aggregate value, the value of the life containing these many local pleasures is fixed in comparison with competing forms of life, and so the finally effective magnitudes are fixed by global desires." My point is that a cow is incapable of having the requisite global desires.

states, the air of mystery is dispelled. For there is nothing odd about the suggestion that a relation obtaining between momentary states of a cow cannot obtain between sequences of those states. One moment can be better or worse for a cow than another moment, but one sequence of moments cannot be better for a cow than another sequence, because a cow cannot care about extended periods in its life. This conclusion seems mysterious only if we imagine one moment as better for the cow than another by virtue of containing more of a special stuff that cannot help but accumulate.

For a lower animal, then, momentary well-being fails not only of additivity but of cumulability by any algorithm at all. Consequently, the totality of this subject's life simply has no value for him, because he cannot care about it as such, and because its constituent moments, which he can care about, have values that don't accumulate.

This conception of a lower animal's interests is supported, I think, by its fruitfulness in accounting for our intuitions about the moral difference between killing animals and killing people. For in relation to an animal's interests, as I have now described them, the traditional Epicurean arguments about death are correct. That is, there is no moment at which a cow can be badly off because of death, since where death is, the cow isn't; and if there is no moment at which a cow is harmed by death, then it cannot be harmed by death at all. A premature death doesn't rob the cow of the chance to accumulate more momentary well-being, since momentary well-being isn't cumulable for a cow; nor can a premature death detract from the value of the cow's life as a whole, since a cow has no interest in its life as a whole, being unable to care about what sort of life it lives.

Of course, a person can care about what his life story is like, and a premature death can spoil the story of his life. Hence, death can harm a person, but it cannot harm a cow.[48]

---

48 Here I am not saying that a premature death is bad for a person because he wants or would want his life to be longer. Rather, I am saying that because a person can want his life to be longer, the judgment that a premature death is bad for him satisfies the requirements of internalism. To cite a person's actual or potential desires as evidence that a value judgment is compatible with internalism is one thing; to cite those desires as the value judgment's truth-makers is quite another. These brief remarks on the evil of death were inspired by Thomas Nagel's essay "Death", in *Mortal Questions*, pp. 1-10. Nagel points out that the Epicurean argument assumes that if death harms its victim, it must harm him at a particular time. Nagel argues that this assumption is false. (So does Fred Feldman, in "Some Puzzles About the Evil of Death".) My claim is that although the assumption is indeed false in application to persons (which is the application that Nagel has in mind), it is true in application to lower animals.

8. So It Goes[1]

Change presupposes a certain position which I take up and from which I see things in procession before me: there are no events without someone to whom they happen and whose finite perspective is the basis of their individuality. Time presupposes a view of time. It is, therefore, not like a river, not a flowing substance. The fact that the metaphor based on this comparison has persisted from the time of Heraclitus to our own day is explained by our surreptitiously putting into the river a witness of its course. … Time is, therefore, not a real process, not an actual succession that I am content to record. It arises from my relation to things.

— M. Merleau-Ponty[2]

I believe that the existence of an enduring self is an illusion and that this illusion is the root of the suffering inherent in the human condition. I am not

---

1   This chapter was presented as the first Amherst Lecture in Philosophy on March 9, 2006 and published at http://www.amherstlecture.org/velleman2006/index.html. It was reprinted in *Introduction to Philosophy: Classical and Contemporary Readings*, ed. John Perry, Michael Bratman, and John Martin Fischer (Oxford: Oxford University Press, 2010), pp. 371-382. I am grateful to Amherst College; its philosophy department; and the department's then-chair, Alex George, for organizing the lecture series and inviting me to inaugurate it. The chapter was also presented to the graduate students in philosophy at New York University and to the philosophy departments of Wake Forest University, the Graduate Center at The City University of New York, Dartmouth College, Georgetown University, the University of Melbourne, Monash University, and the Research School of Social Sciences of the Australian National University. The chapter was written during my term as a visiting professor in the philosophy department at the University of North Carolina at Chapel Hill. My visit was funded by a grant from the Mellon Foundation to Susan Wolf. Some of the ideas were developed in a reading group on the metaphysics of time, led by Thomas Hofweber. My thanks go to Susan, Thomas, the Mellon Foundation, and the UNC department for a very stimulating semester. For comments on earlier versions, I am grateful to John Bigelow, Jay Garfield, Thomas Hofweber, Joel Kupperman, Peter Ludlow, and Daniel J. Velleman.
2   Maurice Merleau-Ponty, *Phenomenology of Perception*, trans. Colin Smith (London: Routledge and Kegan Paul, 1962), pp. 411-412.

a scholar of Buddhism or a practitioner, and this lecture is not an exercise in Buddhist studies. I merely want to explore whether this particular Buddhist thought can be understood in terms familiar to analytic philosophy. How might the illusion of an enduring self lie at the root of human suffering?

One of my reasons for wanting to understand this thought is that it challenges an attitude shared by several philosophers who might otherwise seem sympathetic to the Buddhist conception of the self. Philosophers as diverse as Christine Korsgaard and Daniel Dennett have claimed that the self is something that we must invent or construct.[3] But these philosophers believe that inventing or constructing a self is a wonderful accomplishment of which we should be proud, whereas the Buddhists believe that it is a tragic mistake that we should try to undo. Can Western philosophers make sense of the Buddhist attitude? That's what I want to know.

One philosopher who professes to embrace the Buddhist attitude is Derek Parfit, reflecting on his own neo-Lockean theory of personal identity.[4] Locke argued that our past selves are the people whose experiences we remember first-personally. Parfit points out that the experiences of a single person in the past might in principle be remembered by more than one of us in the present — if, for example, the hemispheres of the person's brain had been transplanted into two different bodies. In that case, there would be more than one of us with a claim to a single past self, a situation incompatible with the logic of identity. Hence connections of memory do not necessarily trace out the career of a single, enduring object, and they are unsuited to serve as the integuments of an enduring self.

Parfit suggests that giving up our belief in an enduring self would be beneficial. Of the time when he believed in his own endurance, he says, "I seemed imprisoned in myself":[5]

---

3   See Christine M. Korsgaard, *The Sources of Normativity*, ed. Onora O'Neill (Cambridge: Cambridge University Press, 1996); idem., "Self-Constitution: Action, Identity, and Integrity", The Locke Lectures, 2002; Daniel C. Dennett, "The Origins of Selves", *Cogito* 3 (1989): 163-173; idem., "The Reality of Selves", in *Consciousness Explained* (Boston: Little, Brown and Company, 1991), pp. 412-430; idem., "The Self as the Center of Narrative Gravity", in *Self and Consciousness: Multiple Perspectives*, eds. Frank S. Kessel, Pamela M. Cole, and Dale L. Johnson (Hillsdale, NJ: Erlbaum Associates, 1992), pp. 103-115.

4   One might think that Parfit's arguments militate not just against the self's endurance but also against its persistence in any sense, including perdurance. (For the difference between endurance and perdurance, see below.) But as David Lewis showed, Parfit's arguments do not necessarily militate against perduring selves. (See Lewis, "Survival and Identity", in *The Identities of Persons*, ed. Amélie Oksenberg Rorty [Berkeley, CA: University of California Press, 1976], pp. 17-40, reprinted in *Philosophical Papers*, vol. I [Oxford: Oxford University Press, 1983], pp. 55-77.)

5   Derek Parfit, *Reasons and Persons* (Oxford: Oxford University Press, 1984), p. 281.

My life seemed like a glass tunnel, through which I was moving faster every year, and at the end of which there was darkness. When I changed my view, the walls of my glass tunnel disappeared. I now live in the open air.

Parfit elsewhere describes this liberation in less metaphorical terms:[6]

Egoism, the fear not of near but of distant death, the regret that so much of one's only life should have gone by — these are not, I think, wholly natural or instinctive. They are all strengthened by the beliefs about personal identity which I have been attacking. If we give up these beliefs, they should be weakened.

Parfit explicitly notes the similarity between his view of personal identity and that of the Buddhists,[7] but he does not directly compare the consolations claimed for these views. Such a comparison might have suggested to Parfit that he underestimates the revolution in attitude that his view of personal identity can produce. For he claims that the consolations of his view can be obtained by attending to the philosophical arguments for it,[8] whereas the Buddhists believe that they can be obtained only through long and arduous meditational practice.

I will argue that shedding our belief in an enduring self would have consequences far more radical than Parfit has imagined — results that cannot be obtained by philosophical argument alone. Breaking out of a glass tunnel is not the half of it.

In order to understand how belief in an enduring self could lead to suffering, we have to understand the ontological status of the self believed in. What exactly would it be for the self to endure?

Metaphysicians have defined two distinct conceptions of how objects persist through time.[9] Under one conception, objects are extended in time as they are extended in space. Just as a single point in space can contain only part of an extended object, a spatial part, so a single point in time can contain only part of a persisting object, a temporal part. The object fills time by having one temporal part after another, just as it fills space by having

---

6   Parfit, "Personal Identity", *The Philosophical Review* 80 (1971): 27.

7   See Parfit, *Reasons and Persons*, pp. 273, 280, 502-503.

8   Ibid., p. 280.

9   See Sally Haslanger, "Persistence Through Time", in *The Oxford Handbook of Metaphysics*, ed. Michael J. Loux and Dean W. Zimmerman (Oxford: Oxford University Press, 2005), pp. 315-354.

one spatial part next to another. An object that persists through time in this way is said to *perdure*.

Under the alternative conception, an object's extension in time is different from its extension in space. Whereas only part of an object can be present at a single point in space, the object can be wholly present at a single point in time. An object that persists through time in this way is said to *endure*.

But what does it mean to say that the object is wholly present at a single point in time?[10] To be sure, all of its spatial parts can be present at a single instant, but all of its spatial parts are conceived to be simultaneously present under the conception of it as perduring, too. And saying that the object is wholly present at a single point in time cannot mean that all of its *temporal* parts are present. For how can all of the object's temporal parts be present at a single point in time if the object also exists at other times?

According to some philosophers, saying that an object is wholly present at a single point in time means that it does not have temporal parts at all. Yet what is to prevent us from considering the object as it is at a single moment and then denominating that aspect of it as a temporal part? If the object is extended in some dimension such as time, and that dimension is itself divisible into smaller and smaller regions, such as hours and minutes and seconds, then nothing can prevent us from abstracting temporal parts from the object by prescinding from its existence beyond one of those regions. The nature of endurance thus appears mysterious. And the suspicion arises that we couldn't possibly believe in an enduring self, because we have no coherent idea what it would be for the self to endure.

These brief considerations fall far short of proving that no coherent idea of an enduring self can be found. But rather than pursue a coherent idea of an enduring self, we should consider the possibility that an incoherent idea will do. An incoherent idea will certainly do if the enduring self is just an illusion. Maybe if we figure out how such an illusion might arise, we will understand the resulting idea, coherent or not.

In my view, the idea of an enduring self arises from the structure of experience and experiential memory, just as Locke first suggested.[11] When I

---

10 The following objections to the traditional conception of endurance are developed more fully in Thomas Hofweber and J. David Velleman, "How to Endure", *The Philosophical Quarterly* 61 (2011): 37-57. These objections would not apply under the theory of time known as presentism. I discuss presentism briefly below.

11 This paragraph and the four that follow summarize a lengthy argument presented in my "Self to Self", *The Philosophical Review* 105 (1996): 39-76; reprinted in *Self to Self: Selected*

remember a past experience, I remember the world as experienced from the perspective of a past self. My memory has an egocentric representational scheme, centered on the person who originally had the experience from which the memory is derived. That person's standpoint lies at a spatiotemporal distance from the present standpoint that I occupy while entertaining the memory. But the mind is not especially scrupulous about the distinction between the subjects occupying these distinct points of view.

Consider, for example, my memory of blowing out the candles on a particular birthday cake in 1957. This memory includes an experiential image of a cake and candles as seen by a five-year-old boy. Now, if I invite you to imagine that you are that birthday boy, then you will conjure up a similar image in your imagination. You might report this thought experiment by saying, "I've just imagined that I am the birthday boy at David Velleman's fifth birthday party." The first occurrence of the pronoun 'I' in this report would of course refer to you, whoever you are: let's say you're Jane Doe. But what about the second occurrence of 'I'? Have you imagined that you, Jane Doe, are the birthday boy? Surely, you haven't imagined a bizarre scenario in which the five-year-old David Velleman is somehow identical with a completely unrelated woman (as we are supposing) named Jane Doe. Rather, you have simply imagined *being* the five-year-old David Velleman, by imagining the birthday party as experienced by him.[12] You have formed an experiential image whose content might be summed up by the statement "I am the birthday boy" as uttered in the imagined scene by the five-year-old David Velleman — a statement in which 'I' would refer to him, the one experiencing the scene, rather than you, the one who has imagined it.[13] When you say, "I've imagined that I am the birthday boy," you should be interpreted as saying, "I've imagined an experience with the content 'I am the birthday boy'," or "I've imagined 'I am the birthday boy'," where the first occurrence of 'I' refers to you but the second refers to him.

Essays (Cambridge: Cambridge University Press, 2005), pp. 170-202. See also "The Identity Problem", part 1 of chapter 6 in this volume.

12 This point was made by Bernard Williams in "Imagination and the Self", in *Problems of the Self: Philosophical Papers 1956–1972* (Cambridge: Cambridge University Press, 1973), pp. 26-45. I discuss Williams's paper in "Self to Self".

13 The second 'I' functions as what Héctor-Neri Castañeda called a quasi-indicator — a pronoun in indirect discourse that takes the place of what was a first-personal pronoun in direct discourse. For an explanation of quasi-indicators (clearer than Castañeda's), see John Perry, "Belief and Acceptance", in *The Problem of the Essential Indexical and Other Essays* (New York: Oxford University Press, 1993), pp. 53-68.

What then of my experiential memory? When I say, "I remember that I was the birthday boy," I am making a report similar to yours. That is, I am reporting an experiential memory whose content would be expressed by the statement "I am the birthday boy" as uttered in the remembered scene by the five-year-old who experienced it. But whereas you may be aware that you haven't imagined the birthday boy's being you, Jane Doe, I am strongly inclined to think that I have remembered his being me, the present subject of this memory.[14] I thereby conflate my remembering self with the self of the experience remembered. When I say, "I remember that I was the birthday boy," I take myself to be referring twice to my present self. I who remember the experience and the "I" of the experience thus become superimposed, so that a single self appears to be present in both.

The selves superimposed in this appearance are two momentary subjects: I in my present capacity as the subject of memory, existing just in the moment of remembering; and the "I" of the remembered experience, who existed just in the moment of the experience. In either case, I am conceived as wholly present at a single point in time, either as me-here-and-now, entertaining the memory, or as "me"-there-and-then, having the experience. Superimposing one of these momentary subjects on the other yields the illusion that they are numerically identical — that the subject whose existence was complete in the moment of the experience

---

14 But isn't it a contingent truth-condition of my memory that the remembered experience has been undergone by me rather than someone else? And if so, how can the second 'I' in "I remember that I was the birthday boy" refer merely to the subject of the remembered experience, who necessarily did undergo it, if anyone did? The answer is that the memory refers to the subject of the remembered experience indexically, pointing to him at the perspectival point of origin in the remembered experience, by pointing to him at the corresponding point in my memory-image, which purports to be a copy derived from that experience. If the image is indeed a copy derived from an experience, as it purports to be, then indexical reference to the "me" of that experience succeeds, and his being the birthday boy is what I veridically remember; if the image is not copied from an experience, then its indexical reference to the "me" of that experience fails — it refers to no one at all — and the memory is illusory. In order for the memory to be veridical, then, the remembered experience must have been undergone by me in the sense that its subject must be accessible to indexical reference as "me".

Of course, your image of being my five-year-old self also refers to the birthday boy as "me", but not in the same, genuinely indexical way. In conjuring up this image, you had to stipulate that its point of origin is occupied by the five-year-old David Velleman, thus referring to him by name before you could go on to think of him as "me". In remembering the experience, I can refer to him as "me" directly, without any stipulation about whom the pronoun refers to, relying on the causal history of my image to secure my reference to the original subject. That is the sense in which I have first-personal access to him whereas you do not. (For further discussion of this issue, see "Self to Self" and "The Identity Problem".)

remembered was one and the same as the subject whose existence is complete in the moment of remembering. This appearance is already incoherent if one and the same thing cannot have its existence confined to each of two different moments. The incoherence is compounded by the thought that this momentary subject has persisted through the interval between the original experience and the memory, existing in its entirety at each intervening moment.[15]

The same effect is produced by experiential anticipation, in which I prefigure a future experience from the perspective that I expect to occupy in it. A single self appears to have its full existence both now and later, because I who anticipate the experience and the "I" of the anticipated experience become superimposed.

For a spatial analog of the resulting idea, think of the scene in which Woody Allen plays a spermatozoon about to be launched from the loins of … Woody Allen.[16] In reality, of course, a person occupies different points in space with different parts of himself, none of which is identical to any other part or to the person as a whole. We might say, then, that a person *pervades* space. In this scene, however, Woody Allen occupies different points in space with a smaller self that plays the role of each spatial part of his own body. We might say, then, that he *invades* space rather than pervading it. Incoherent, to say the least. Yet experiential memory leads me to think that my own temporal extension is composed of a single momentary self playing the role of each temporal part of my existence.

I am tempted to say that all of my temporal parts are present at a single point in time because I tend to think of myself as my present self — a momentary subject whose existence is indeed complete in the here-and-now. I am tempted to say that I nevertheless persist through time because I tend to think of this self, complete in the moment, as nevertheless existing at other moments. And because I therefore conceive of each moment in my

---

15 I find indirect evidence for these claims about autobiographical memory in the experience of reading truly gifted autobiographical novelists, such as Laura Ingalls Wilder (*Little House on the Prairie*) or Elspeth Huxley (*The Flame Trees of Thika*). These authors were able to depict past experience as it was registered by the childish minds of their younger selves. Reading their work, I am struck by the contrast with my own childhood memories, in which the psychological distance between the mind that stored a memory and the mind that retrieves it is foreshortened, so that past experience seems to have been registered by my current, adult consciousness — the remembering "I", who has been superimposed on the "I" remembered.

16 In *Everything You Always Wanted to Know About Sex* But Were Afraid to Ask*, dir. Woody Allen, Rollins-Joffe Productions, United Artists, 1972.

temporal extension as containing my complete self, I am tempted to deny that it contains a mere temporal part of me. There I am, all of me, at my fifth birthday party; here I am, all of me, remembering that party; there I will be, all of me, on my seventy-fifth birthday — as if one and the same momentary subject can play the several parts of my five-year-old, sixty-two-year-old, and seventy-five-year-old selves. I think of myself as all of me, all the time, just as Woody Allen is all Woody Allen in every one of his cells.

What would be the consequences of truly shedding our sense of being enduring objects and learning to conceive of ourselves as perduring instead? I want to suggest that the existence of an enduring self, if it is indeed an illusion, is one of two illusions that go hand-in-hand. A consequence of shedding the one illusion would be to shed the other as well. The other illusion of which I speak has to do with the nature of time.

The concept of perdurance for objects is most at home in a conception of time known as eternalism. According to eternalists, all of the temporal facts can be expressed in terms of the temporal relations between events. One event can occur earlier or later than another, or simultaneously, and it can be closer to or further from the other in time. The relations among events as earlier, later, or simultaneous, and closer or further apart, exhaust the temporal facts, in the eyes of eternalists: there is no more to time than these relations.

The philosopher J. Ellis McTaggart argued that the temporal relations among events are not sufficient to satisfy our concept of time, although he also argued that the concept is incoherent.[17] Temporal relations among events do not change, and so McTaggart argued that they cannot account for the passage of time — that is, for the way events draw nearer from the future, until they occur in the present and, having occurred, recede into the past. When we say that a future event is always drawing closer and closer, eternalists must understand us as meaning only that the event is nearer to our second utterance of the word 'closer' than it was to the first. And these temporal relations are as they always were and always will be; or, rather, they exist timelessly, constituting time itself. The future event that we describe as drawing closer and closer not only stands closer to the last word of our description than it does to the earlier words; it always has and always will stand in those relations, or it stands in them timelessly. Such

---

17 J. Ellis McTaggart, "The Unreality of Time", *Mind* 17 (1908): 457-474.

unchanging relations cannot constitute time, McTaggart argued, because time requires change — specifically, the change that consists in an event's approaching from the future, arriving in the present, and receding into the past.

Yet the change thus required by our concept of time struck McTaggart as paradoxical and hence impossible. An event's changing from future to present to past must unfold *in time*: the event must be first in the future, then in the present, and then again in the past. And having added these temporal indices ("first", "then", "then again") to our description of the change, we have reverted to an eternalist idiom. We have said that the event's status as a future event occurs first — that is, earlier than its status as present and past; that its status as present occurs later than its status as future; and that its status as past occurs even later than the other two. Thus, in order to complete our description of how time passes, we have been forced to describe it once again in terms of those temporal relations which never change.

There is a temptation to say, at this point, that what moves is not the future or past but the present, or rather the property of being the present, which belongs successively to different sets of events. But if we try to describe how the property of being present passes from one set of events to the next, we will end up saying that it belongs first to one set, then to another, and then again to a third, as they occur in succession. We will thereupon have said no more than this: that the property of being present belongs earlier to some events than to others, always belonging to events simultaneously with their occurrence. So in what sense can the present be said to move? Every event is present sooner or later, and that fact never changes.

One fairly desperate attempt to solve the problem is a theory known as presentism. According to presentism, only the present exists; past and future are merely tenses modifying facts about the present.[18]

Presentism is best explained by an analogy between time and modality. Consider the fact that John Kerry might have won the 2004 presidential election. We could restate this fact by saying that a Kerry victory occurs in a merely possible history, alternative to the one that actually unfolded in 2004; but perhaps we wouldn't then be speaking with metaphysical

---

18 In the following paragraphs I have drawn on John Bigelow, "The Passage of Time" (MS).

strictness. Perhaps we should acknowledge only one event — Kerry's loss, which actually occurred — plus the subjunctively statable fact, also true of actuality, that Kerry might have won instead. According to this view, called actualism, there is no Kerry victory that occurs in a realm of mere possibility: actual events are the only events there are.[19]

Presentism goes one step further, refusing to acknowledge even an event of Kerry's losing the election. For when we describe Kerry's loss as occurring in the past, the presentist claims that we are speaking just as loosely as we would in describing his victory as occurring in some alternative possible history. The only events there are, according to the presentist, are the ones occurring now in actuality. Just as Kerry's possibly having won is a fact about actuality, statable in the subjunctive, so his previously having lost is a fact about the present, statable in the past tense. That he might have won, and that he did lose, are subjunctive and past-tense facts about the actual present, which is all there is for facts to be about. There is no Kerry victory occurring in a realm of possibility; and there is not even a Kerry loss occurring in a realm of the past.

The presentist claims that his view enables us to represent the passage of time. The occurrence of an event entails the fact that it will have occurred, and hence that it will later be a matter of past-tense fact. (More precisely, the event's occurrence entails the future-tense fact that there will be a past-tense fact of its having occurred.) This entailment is said to represent the passage of the event from the present into the past. The occurrence of an event is also incompatible with the fact that it wasn't going to occur, and compatible with the fact that it was going to occur. Hence its present occurrence entails that it was previously a subject of future-tense facts, an entailment that is said to represent its passage from the future into the present. Finally, the occurrence of an event is compatible with its being the case neither that the event was going to occur nor that it wasn't going to, while nevertheless entailing that the event definitely will have occurred. That is, while there previously may have been no fact of the matter whether the event would occur, there will later be a determinate fact of its having occurred — a constellation of facts that is said to represent how an open future gets closed up into a fixed past.[20]

---

19 So-called modal realists, such as David Lewis, believe that there are events and things inhabiting such a realm, but the intuitions of most philosophers run to the contrary.

20 That there was previously no fact of the matter whether the event would occur, and that there will later be a determinate fact of its having occurred, are of course past- and future-tense facts about the present, according to presentism. The same goes for all of the entailments discussed in this paragraph.

The presentist also claims that his view enables us to solve our problem about the concept of endurance. Just as there is no John Kerry existing in an alternative possible history in which he won the election, according to presentism, so there is no John Kerry existing in a past in which he lost: all there is of John Kerry is the present John Kerry. This person has the past-tense properties of having existed in 2004 and having lost the election of that year, just as he has the subjunctive property that he might have won; but the presentist insists that these properties belong to Kerry's actual present self, which is all of him that exists. Hence, the presentist can deny that John Kerry perdures, by denying that he has any temporal parts. According to presentism, Kerry's existence is confined to the present.

One drawback of presentism is that it requires the present to bear sufficient features to render true not only present-tense facts but all past-tense facts as well: the present must, as it were, bear witness to all of history.[21] A more serious problem, for my purposes, is that presentism doesn't really solve the problems of endurance and the passage of time. What presentism describes is — not a changing prospect in which events approach from the future, arrive in the present, and recede into the past — but a single, static structure of past-prospective and future-perfect facts, all true of the present. Tensed facts about the present entail other tensed facts about the present, but nothing moves. Similarly, presentism describes objects as being wholly present at every moment of their existence, but only because it describes them as existing at only one moment, the present; and so it describes them as enduring in only a trivial sense. According to presentism, objects have past- and future-tensed properties, but the objects themselves exist only in the present, and so they don't persist at all, much less endure.

Surely, we should hope for a more intuitively satisfying solution to the problems of endurance and temporal passage. I think that the solution is to recognize that both phenomena are illusions, and that these illusions are interdependent. I have already suggested how the illusion of an enduring self might arise from the structure of first-personal memory and anticipation. I will now suggest that the illusion of an enduring self gives rise to another illusion: that of movement with respect to time.

Our difficulty in characterizing such movement was that, when we tried to identify something toward which a future event draws nearer or from

---

21 For this objection, see Simon Keller, "Presentism and Truthmaking", in *Oxford Studies in Metaphysics*, vol. I, ed. Dean W. Zimmerman (Oxford: Oxford University Press, 2004), pp. 83-106 (cited by Bigelow).

which a past event recedes, we focused our attention on other events. Yet each event depends for its identity on when it occurs: it could not be closer to a future event, or further from a past event, without occupying a different temporal position and hence being a different event. This conception of the problem suggests the solution. Whatever the future draws nearer to, or the past recedes from, must be something that can exist at different positions in time with its identity intact. And we have already found such a thing — or the illusion of one, at least — in the form of the enduring self.

Suppose that I endure in the admittedly incoherent sense that is suggested by experiential memory and anticipation. In that case, I exist in my entirety at successive moments in time, thereby moving in my entirety with respect to events. As I move through time, future events draw nearer to me and past events recede. Time truly passes, in the sense that it passes *me*.

If I merely perdure, however, then I do not move with respect to time. I extend through time with newer and newer temporal parts, but all of my parts remain stationary. A perduring self can be compared to a process, such as the performance of a symphony. The performance doesn't move with respect to time; it merely extends newer and newer temporal parts to fill each successive moment. The last note of the performance is of course closer to midnight than the first, but we wouldn't say that midnight and the performance move closer together. Midnight is separated from the performance by a timelessly fixed but extremely vague interval, which can be made precise only with respect to particular parts of the performance — the first note, the second note, the third note — each of which is separated from midnight by an interval that is also timelessly fixed. Similarly, we wouldn't say that the ceiling and I get closer together from my feet to my head. The ceiling stands above me at a fixed but vague distance, which can be made precise only with respect to particular parts of me — feet, waist, head — each of which is separated from it by a fixed distance.

But if I am an enduring thing, then midnight and I get closer together, and not just in the sense that I extend temporal parts closer to it than my earlier parts. I don't just extend from a 9:00 p.m. stage to a 10:00 p.m. stage that is closer to midnight, as I extend from my feet to a head that is closer to the ceiling; I exist in my entirety within the stroke of 9:00, and I exist again within the stroke of 10:00 — the selfsame entity twice, existing once further from midnight and then all over again, closer. Midnight occupies two different distances from my fully constituted self. From my perspective, then, midnight draws nearer.

If this enduring "me" is an illusion, however, then so is the passage of time. And ceasing to think of myself as an enduring subject should result in my ceasing to experience the passage of time. Coming to think of myself as perduring should result in my coming to experience different temporal parts of myself at different moments, but no enduring self past which those moments can flow.

Suppose that I could learn to experience my successive moments of consciousness — *now* and *now* and *now* — as successive notes in a performance with no enduring listener, no self-identical subject for whom these moments would be *now* and *then* and *then again*. In remembering a scene that I experienced in the past, I would distinguish between the "I" who remembers it and the "I" who experienced it; in anticipating a scene that I would experience in the future, I would distinguish between the anticipating "I" and the experiencing "I" as well. Hence, my present self would be cognizant of being distinct from the past subjects from whom it receives memories and the future subjects for whom it stores up anticipations. It would therefore have no conception of a single subject to which events could bear different relations over time, nothing to which they could draw near or from which they could recede. It would think of itself, and each of the subjects with whom it communicates by memory and anticipation, as seeing its own present moment, with none of them seeing a succession of moments as present.

The result would be that time would no longer seem to pass, because my experience would no longer include a subject of its passage — just successive momentary subjects, each timelessly entrenched in its own temporal perspective. I would think of myself as filling time rather than passing through it or having it pass me by — as existing in time the way a rooted plant exists in space, growing extensions to occupy it without moving in relation to it. Having shed the illusion of an enduring self, I would have lost any sense of time as passing at all.

One small bit of evidence in support of this speculation is that when I lose awareness of myself, by "losing myself" in engrossing activities, I also tend to lose awareness of time's passing.[22] With my attention fully devoted

---

22 See Mihaly Csikszentmihalyi, *Flow: The Psychology of Optimal Experience* (New York: Harper & Row, 1990). According to Csikszentmihalyi, losing awareness of self and losing awareness of time are two of the characteristic features of "flow" experiences. I discuss these experiences further in "What Good is a Will?", in *Action in Context*, ed. Anton Leist (Berlin: Walter de Gruyter, 2007); and "The Way of the Wanton", in *Practical Identity and Narrative Agency*, ed. Kim Atkins and Catriona MacKenzie (London: Routledge, 2008),

to playing a sport, reading a book, writing a paragraph, I am drawn out of myself and, as it seems, out of the passage of time as well. Conversely, when I have nothing to occupy my attention — that is, when I am bored — my attention returns to myself, and the passage of time becomes painfully salient. Self-awareness and time-awareness thus seem to go hand-in-hand.

Clearly, I am nowhere near to "losing myself" in this way on a lasting basis, despite being convinced, by the arguments of Locke and Parfit, that I am in fact a perduring rather than an enduring self. Truly assimilating the implications of those arguments would entail radical changes in my experience, changes of the sort that no argument can produce. No wonder the Buddhists believe that dispelling the illusion of an enduring self requires an arduous regimen of meditation.

As we have seen, Parfit blames our belief in an enduring self for emotions that might well be the essence of our existential suffering: grief over time past and anxiety at the prospect of death. Parfit suggests that these emotions get their sting from our proprietary interest in our one and only life — that glass tunnel in which we imagine ourselves to be enclosed, when we believe that we have enduring selves. Parfit claims to derive consolation from shedding this belief because he no longer views his relation to the person lost in the past, or to the person who will die in the future, as a relation of identity. The consolation comes when he escapes from seeming imprisoned in an enduring self.

Yet I don't see why bearing a less robust relation to his own past and future is any consolation to Parfit. Why should a sense of partial alienation from past and future selves leave him feeling relieved rather than bereft? It's not as if he has come to realize that this isn't his "only life"; he has merely come to realize that it isn't even *his* in the sense that he previously thought. This realization provides only the cold comfort of having nothing to lose.

When Parfit describes the drawbacks of believing in an enduring self, he speaks not only about the loneliness of proprietorship in a single life — being imprisoned in a glass tunnel — but also about the emotions attendant upon time's passage. He complains of the sense that he is "moving faster and faster" through the tunnel, toward the "darkness" at its end, and of the sense that "so much of one's *only* life should have gone by". Surely, the

---

pp. 169-192; both reprinted in *The Possibility of Practical Reason*, second edition (Ann Arbor, MI: Maize Books, 2015).

remedy for these anxieties and regrets is not to get out of the tunnel and live "in the open air"; the remedy is to *stop moving*.

The remedy for Parfit's distress, in other words, is to become an eternalist. Consider: [23]

> [W]hen a person dies he only appears to die. He is still very much alive in the past, so it is very silly for people to cry at his funeral. All moments, past, present, and future, always have existed, always will exist. ... It is just an illusion ... that one moment follows another one, like beads on a string, and that once a moment is gone is it gone forever.

The speaker here is Billy Pilgrim, relating what he learned on the planet Tralfamadore, where he was once on display as an intergalactic zoological specimen:

> When a Tralfamadorian sees a corpse, all he thinks is that the dead person is in bad condition in that particular moment, but that the same person is just fine in plenty of other moments. Now, when I myself hear that somebody is dead, I simply shrug and say what the Tralfamadorians say about dead people, which is "So it goes."

The Tralfamadorians are eternalists about time, and they have managed to derive great comfort from this philosophy.

Note, however, that whereas Parfit has overcome the illusion of an enduring self but not the illusion of time's passing, the Tralfamadorians have done the reverse: they have overcome the illusion of time's passing, but they still speak as if they believe in an enduring self.[24] This incomplete disillusionment is just as unsatisfactory, to my way of thinking, as Parfit's. Parfit and the Tralfamadorians have divided between them what is a larger truth: the enduring self and the passage of time are interdependent illusions. The Tralfamadorian half of the truth is more consoling than Parfit's, to my mind; but taken by itself, the Tralfamadorian half of the truth is unstable.

The Tralfamadorians speak as if they occupy moments in time with their entire selves, not just temporal parts. Regarding themselves as enduring

---

23 Kurt Vonnegut, Jr., *Slaughterhouse-Five or, The Children's Crusade: A Duty-Dance with Death* (New York: Dell Publishing, 1969), p. 23.

24 But: "Tralfamadorians don't see human beings as two-legged creatures, either. They see them as great millepedes — 'with babies' legs at one end and old people's legs at the other,' says Billy Pilgrim" (ibid., p. 75). This suggests that Tralfamadorians see people as perduring space-time worms rather than enduring objects. Nevertheless, their first-personal descriptions of their own experiences sound like those of an enduring self.

objects, they manage to deny the passage of time only by asserting that they can stand outside of time and range across it at will:

> The Tralfamadorians can look at the different moments just the way we can look at a stretch of the Rocky Mountains, for instance. They can see how permanent all the moments are, and they can look at any moment that interests them.

Billy Pilgrim never fully attains the Tralfamadorian view of time, but he does lose the normal human view: [25]

> Billy Pilgrim has come unstuck in time.
> Billy has gone to sleep a senile widower and awakened on his wedding day. He has walked through a door in 1955 and come out another one in 1941. He has seen his birth and death many times, he says, and pays random visits to all the events in between.
> He says.
> Billy is spastic in time, has no control over where he is going next, and the trips aren't necessarily fun. He is in a constant state of stage fright, he says, because he never knows what part of his life he is going to have to act in next.

How do the Tralfamadorians manage to visit different moments in time, betaking their complete selves from one moment to another? This process would require a higher temporal order of "first" and "later" within which the desultory visits could occur, and across which the Tralfamadorians would retain their identities. A Tralfamadorian's visits to random moments in ordinary time would themselves have to occur at well-ordered moments in a meta-time, which would constitute a temporal stream washing over the Tralfamadorians as relentlessly as ordinary time washes over us. Similarly, Billy Pilgrim is washed by a stream of meta-moments ordering his visits to random moments of ordinary time.

In short, "coming unstuck in time" is not as easy as it sounds. Billy Pilgrim may jump around in one temporal order, but he moves through another in sequence. Escaping the passage of time would require the dissolution of his enduring self. In order to come completely unstuck in time, Billy himself would have to come unglued.

Although the tale of Billy Pilgrim gives a partial and imperfect portrait of life without the illusion of temporal passage, it seems correct in portraying

---

25 Ibid., p. 20.

that life as lacking many of our ordinary worries about mortality. Even so, not all such worries would disappear along with the passage of time.

Billy describes the Tralfamadorians as unconcerned about *being dead*. But of course Epicurus long ago taught us that being dead is nothing — literally — and hence that it is nothing to worry about. The anxiety that makes sense, at least for those of us who live with temporal passage, is anxiety about the inexorable approach of death, about time's *running out*. This anxiety would be allayed if time no longer seemed to pass. And once time no longer seemed to pass, the mere fact of our mortality would no longer seem regrettable. When time seems to be running out, we wish for immortality, which would amount to having infinite time left on the clock. But in an eternalist world, immortality would amount instead to a kind of temporal ubiquity — existing at every future moment. Having an infinite amount time left seems desirable if time is running out; but if time is standing still, then filling an infinite amount of it might well seem unattractive.

Still, those of us who die young could continue to lament the truncated extent of our lives: having too short a life would still be grounds for unhappiness. What would be groundless is unhappiness about mortality itself — the unhappiness that affects everyone, no matter how long-lived, at the sound of death's approaching tread.

Would liberation from the passage of time free us from other kinds of suffering? It certainly wouldn't spare us from physical pain or other unpleasant experiences. But it just might prevent pain and unpleasantness from being transformed into suffering.

We can undergo pain or unpleasantness without suffering under it: suffering is a particular way of experiencing pain or unpleasantness — specifically, of *not coping* with it.[26] And I suspect, though I cannot argue here, that the way of not coping that's constitutive of suffering results from the perception of time as passing. What undoes us, when we suffer with pain, is panic at the thought that it will never abate, that no end is in sight. Patients can learn to bear pain by "accepting" or "being with" it, focusing on the pain of the moment, without thinking about what's next.[27] It's not

---

26 I discuss this conception of suffering in "Beyond Price", chapter 4 in this volume; and "The Gift of Life", part II of chapter 6.

27 Here I am merely gesturing at a large and controversial research program. For just one example, see Lance M. McCracken and Christopher Eccleston, "Coping or Acceptance: What to Do About Chronic Pain?", *Pain* 105 (2003): 197-204; and Lance M. McCracken, James W. Carson, Christopher Eccleston, and Francis J. Keefe, "Acceptance and Change

the pain they're in that makes them suffer but the prospect of its endlessly going on.

Perhaps, then, liberation from the passage of time would entail liberation from suffering altogether, though not, of course, from pain. There would be bad moments and good moments, but no panic about the coming moments, and hence no suffering.

The Tralfamadorians express the consolations of their perspective by saying, "So it goes." Come to think of it, though, the point of this motto is less than obvious. After all, the Tralfamadorians inhabit a perspective in which "it" doesn't "go" at all, since they do not experience time as passing. Why do they say "So it goes"? Why don't they say "So it is"?

Maybe the Tralfamadorian motto has been translated in a manner suitable to us, who simply cannot escape from the illusion of time's passing. "So it goes" means "so it goes *for you*." They are recommending the attitude that is appropriate for creatures who can't help but experience time as passing. Buddhism must offer similar advice, exported not from one planet to another but from the meditative state to the state of ordinary consciousness. What is the appropriate attitude to have in ordinary life, where the self unavoidably seems to endure and time unavoidably seems to pass, given that both appearances are illusions?

I think that the exportable lessons here must include something about the way we cope with the passage of time. We can't stop the self from seeming to endure, or stop time from seeming to pass, but we can cope with these phenomena better, given the knowledge that they are merely phenomenal.

Ordinarily I cope rather badly with temporal passage and personal endurance. I don't exactly live in state of Pilgrim-esque stage fright, continually unsure when I might find myself at my fifth birthday party or my seventy-fifth. In some respects, I feel like a Tralfamadorian, because I can choose which parts of my life to visit, in memory and anticipation. Yet I have a disconcerting tendency to live different parts of my life all at once — to relive the past and pre-live the future even while I'm trying to live in

---

in the Context of Chronic Pain", *Pain* 109 (2004): 4-7. One of the methods discussed in the latter article is "Mindfulness-Based Stress Reduction", which is described as "moment-to-moment observation and acceptance of the continually changing reality of the present" (5). For some of the methodological problems in this area, see Christopher Eccleston, "The Attentional Control of Pain: Methodological and Theoretical Concerns", *Pain* 63 (1995): 3-10.

the present. And even as I relive my past in a memory, it is at the same time slipping away from me, as there comes bearing down on me a future that I am pre-living in anticipation.

It's as if too many parts of my life are on the table at once, and yet somehow they are continually being served up and snatched away like dishes in a restaurant whose waitstaff is too impatient to let me eat. And this whole grief- and anxiety-provoking conception of my life has been adopted out of panic over the passage of time, which requires me to anticipate the future precisely because it's bearing down on me, and to remember the past precisely because it's slipping away.

Once I know that the self doesn't endure, and time doesn't pass, then even when under the illusion to the contrary, I can better follow the Buddhist injunction to be fully aware of the present moment. The realization that I am *of* the moment — that is, a momentary part of a temporally extended self — can remind me to be *in* the moment, which draws my attention away from time's passage, even if it doesn't succeed it stopping time from seeming to pass. Insofar as I can be in the moment, I can perhaps gain some respite from the grief and anxiety of that overwhelmed diner, on whom loaded plates are bearing down even as uneaten dishes are being borne away. Each moment can be devoted to savoring the dish of the moment.

9. Dying[1]

Some people hope to die in their sleep. Not me. I don't regret having been oblivious at my birth, but I don't want to be napping at my death.

My birth hasn't figured much in my life, other than having begun it, whereas my death will have figured far more than just ending it. It's been on my mind, one way or another, ever since I learned what death is. I've wondered about it, worried about it, once or twice wished for it, and in any case constantly sensed its presence in my future.

One usually thinks of death in the abstract. But at some point it dawned on me that I will have a particular death, my very own death. Since that moment of clarity, I have felt possessive about my death. Death is a momentous life event, and I am going to get one.

The expectation of getting a death of one's own lies behind the ancient belief in the Fates.

They are the guardians of the tantalizing facts as to when, where, and how one will die, the facts that will finally bring the abstraction of death down to earth. We have dispensed with the Fates but not with their function; we've merely reassigned it to the cardiologists and oncologists. They tell us the "how" of our deaths, and then we demand the "when" by asking, "How long have I got?" Of course, physicians are not the Fates, and trying to cast them in that role introduces unnecessary frustration into the doctor-patient relationship. Having a diagnosis is not enough, but it's all we can get until our fate is revealed by being fulfilled.

1 Originally published in *Think* 11 (2012): 29-32, http://dx.doi.org/10.1017/S14771756120
0022X

Many philosophers think that death is a deprivation, whereas immortality would at worst be a bore. I see deprivation on the side of immortality. Being immortal would entail living forever without life's most persistently anticipated consummation.

Immortality is not a deprivation for the gods, who have known literally forever that they would never die and who have therefore never considered the prospect: the gods have always planned on being immortal. Their immortality is quite different from what mortals would get if granted a reprieve. As nouveaux immortals, human beings would have spent years contemplating their inevitable death only to be told, "Never mind." But I do mind, have minded all of my life with all of my mental strength. At this point, I'd rather go through with it.

Going through with it would be a bad idea if death were a significant harm. But I have lost my grip on the philosophical question about the harm of death. I've lost my grip because I cannot imagine an answer that would affect how I feel about death, and I can't imagine how anything could count as an answer unless it would affect how I feel.[2]

When I say that my feelings wouldn't be affected, I don't mean that they are permanently settled; I mean that they are permanently unsettled. About death, most of us have mixed feelings most of the time.

Our feelings about death are mixed because we see it as the end of our life stories and we can tell those stories, and that ending, in many different ways.[3] We can tell the story of missing out on the future; we can tell the story of running out of time; we can tell the story of becoming nothing but a memory. None of these is a good story, but they are bad in different ways — sad, scary, spooky. And then there are stories that aren't bad at all: the old-time Christian story of laying down our burdens, the Buddhist story of living fully in each one of just so many moments.

What would it mean for one of these stories to be the right one and the others to be wrong?

What would it mean for one of the associated feelings to be right and the others wrong? I don't know; and so I no longer know what's at stake in the philosophical debate about the harm of death.

---

2   For this conception of value, see "Love and Nonexistence", part III of chapter 6 in this volume.

3   For the relation between value and narrative, see "Well-Being and Time", chapter 7 in this volume.

We can, of course, come to realize that we have spun out some of these stories too far. If we imagine that laying down our burdens will lead to a refreshing night's sleep, then we're making a mistake; we're also making a mistake if we imagine that we'll be disappointed at missing out on the future. Yet even after we adjust our stories to the realities of death, the adjusted stories remain compelling: we really will be relieved of our burdens, even if we won't feel the relief; we really will miss out on the future, even if we won't know what we're missing. Nonexistence isn't *that* difficult to comprehend; and no one can tell us that we're mistaken to feel forward-looking relief or forward- looking disappointment about it, despite knowing that we won't feel relief or disappointment at the time.

That said, I have now argued that there's something to be learned — namely, that there's nothing else to be learned. Once we realize that we'll never resolve how to feel about death, we can stop trying to resolve it, stop feeling frustrated about not having resolved it, and hence stop feeling at least one of the things that we currently feel. We can also be less rigid in our remaining feelings, by feeling each of them in the awareness that we can also feel otherwise.

They say that when you face death, your whole life passes before your eyes. Taken literally, the expression is ludicrous. Woody Allen:[4]

> They took my hood off and threw a rope around my neck, and they decided to hang me.
> And suddenly my whole life passed before my eyes. I saw myself as a kid again, in Kansas, going to school, swimming at the swimming hole, and fishing, frying up a mess-o-catfish, going down to the general store, getting a piece of gingham for Emmy-Lou. And I realize it's not my life. They're gonna hang me in two minutes, the wrong life is passing before my eyes.

Having the right life pass before his eyes would not have been as funny, but it would have been just as absurd. A fast-forward replay of his life? With a noose around his neck?

If the expression is to make any sense, it has to mean that when facing death, you suddenly see your life as a completed whole, a particular life bounded at both ends. So long as your life is open-ended, it remains an abstraction, some completion or other of what has gone before. When your

---

4 Woody Allen, "Down South", in *Standup Comic: 1964-1968* (Rhino Records, 1999), CD, http://www.ibras.dk/comedy/allen.htm

life comes to a close, it becomes fully specific and hence concrete. Not to see your life out to its end would be never to have known it as a concrete particular.

In a traditional Jewish wedding, the bride walks around the groom three (or seven) times. As you might expect, there are all sorts of explanations for this custom. I like to think that it gives the bride a good look at what she is getting, not just in the sense of revealing a fat ass but in the sense of showing the groom as a fully specified individual, with all of the details filled in. The bride is being shown that she is marrying a particular man, not an abstraction.

Until people circumnavigated the Earth, they lived somewhere in the midst of somewhere or other. In order to see where they stood, they had to close the circle. Similarly, closing the circle of one's life is necessary to seeing it as the particular life one has lived. And I want to know the particular life I've lived before I stop living it — which will entail fully living it up to the very end.

10. The Rights to a Life[1]

In *After Long Silence,* Helen Fremont tells the story of growing up in the Midwest as the daughter of Polish Catholic parents.[2] She recounts some of the stories they told of their courtship in eastern Poland, which was occupied by the Germans, then occupied by the Soviets — who deported her father to Siberia — and then occupied again by the Germans. She recounts the stories they told of her father's escape back to Poland and, from there, to Rome, where he was reunited with her mother, who had escaped from Poland disguised as an Italian soldier. She recounts the stories they told of their marriage in Rome and eventual emigration to the United States. She tells her own story of growing up in the shadow of her parents' wartime ordeal. She tells the story of coming out as a lesbian to her parents and her Italian aunt.

Helen tells the story of discovering, in her thirties, that her parents were actually Polish Jews — her mother, the daughter of an Orthodox rabbi. She tells the story of gradually uncovering the true history of her parents' separation, escape, and reunification. She recounts that hair-raising history, including all of the cover stories that her mother told in order to elude arrest by the Germans, who had reoccupied eastern Poland; including her mother's new identity as a Polish Catholic girl named Maria, finally married in the Church to her revenant fiancé; including the cover stories that she told to her daughters as a way of fending off their questions about the past.

Helen tells the story of confronting her parents with what she had learned; she tells the story of their initial denials, their sleepless nights of returning memories, their grudging help in her project of reconstructing

---

1   Originally published in *On Life-Writing* (Oxford: Oxford University Press, 2015) edited by Zachary Leader, using a CC BY-NC-ND licence. For permission to reuse this material outside the scope of the CC BY-NC-ND licence, please visit http://www.oup.co.uk/academic/rights/permissions or contact the author.
2   Helen Fremont, *After Long Silence: A Memoir* (New York: Dell Publishing, 1999).

http://dx.doi.org/10.11647/OBP.0061.10

the past. She tells the story of discovering, and then explaining to her mother, how her mother's parents, Helen's grandparents, had died — not "in a bomb", as her mother had always said, but in the gas chambers of Belzec. And, finally, she tells the story of telling all of these stories in a book of which her parents disapproved.

Helen tells these stories in telegraphic, Tralfamadorian style, jumping from wartime Poland, to postwar Italy, to Michigan in the 1950s, to Boston in the 1990s, and back again, unstuck in time.

Helen also enumerates the stories that she cannot tell, because they have been suppressed or repressed or simply forgotten by her parents: she doesn't even know her mother's given name. And in telling the history of her parents' wartime experiences, she deftly hints at the ways in which she is embroidering on shreds of evidence for the sake of telling a good story.

As a child, Helen heard many true stories from her parents and very few lies; they denied their heritage mainly by omission. Did her parents owe her the full story? Was it in any sense her story as well as theirs? What right did Helen have to undo her parents' repression and then to publish their story against their wishes? What right did she have to embellish the story with narrative details that were fictional, despite her insistence that they recreated some narrative truth?

More than most of us, Helen's parents lived through experiences that had the formal structure of a story: meeting and courtship, separation and trials, triumph and reunion: beginning, middle, and end. These events are "their story" in a sense in which their later life in America is not, because the latter doesn't make for a story at all; the former make a story, and it is theirs.

The historiographer Hayden White says that the story form never inheres in events but can only be imposed on them.[3] My view is that the story form is in essence an emotional cadence — an arc of emotions aroused, complicated, and resolved — and I would say that the wartime experiences of Helen's parents had an overall emotional arc of the right shape.[4] These

---

3 For Hayden White on the story form, see *Metahistory: The Historical Imagination in Nineteenth-Century Europe* (Baltimore: Johns Hopkins University Press, 1973); *Tropics of Discourse: Essays in Cultural Criticism* (Baltimore: Johns Hopkins University Press, 1987); and *The Content of Form: Narrative Discourse and Historical Representation* (Baltimore: Johns Hopkins University Press, 1987).

4 I present this analysis of narrative in "Narrative Explanation", *The Philosophical Review* 112 (2003): 1-25. At one point in her book, Helen says, "Something happens, then something happens, then something happens. This is called a story" (p. 247). I disagree.

emotions were the main engines of her parents' progress across Europe, and so the story form really was inherent in their journey.

Helen and her sister were told the outline of this story from their earliest childhood:

> Their love story I had been fed early and often, until it seemed part of my bones. I knew that they had fallen in love before the war, and they had been separated for six years without knowing if the other was alive; my mother escaped Poland dressed as an Italian soldier, and my father walked across Europe after the war, found my mother in Rome, and married her ten years to the day after they had first met. That was the tale they liked to tell and retell, the story they used to summarize their lives. It was a good story, because it ran a thread across the war and connected the two lovers before and after. [p. 8]

Thus, Helen's parents exploited the arc of this story to distract attention from matters unspoken.[5] These matters included facts about the past, but they also included emotions that were very much in the present. Helen says:

> I had been living my life with flawed vision, stumbling in the dark, bumping into things I hadn't realized were there. No one acknowledged anything. Yet each time I walked into my parents' house, I fell over something, or dropped into something, a cavernous silence, an unspoken, invisible danger. [p. 31]

The point of this and similar passages is not that Helen was continually stumbling into the six-year lacuna in her parents' story. There was indeed a narrative lacuna, because narrating those six years would have required her parents to reveal that they were Jewish; but that lacuna is not the "invisible danger" of which Helen speaks here. The invisible danger is not even the danger that her parents faced as Jews in Nazi-occupied Poland. It is rather the danger of unleashing the emotions they retained from that experience. When she says, "No one acknowledged anything," she means that her parents didn't acknowledge the grief and fear they still carried with them. So whereas the often-repeated love story skipped but never falsified facts about the past, it did falsify emotions felt in the present, since their parents were not in fact living happily ever after.

When Helen discovers her Jewish background, she begins attending synagogue, and she eventually seeks instruction in Judaism from a rabbi.

---

5 "The past was always like this, an empty space in our lives, a gap in our conversations, into which our mother tumbled from time to time, quietly, without warning" (p. 145).

There are many reasons why Helen might have tried to enter Judaism, which after all remains foreign to many who identify themselves as Jews. What she suggests is that she was trying to fill out a newfound self-understanding: "All our lives," she tells her mother, "there's been something that just doesn't fit. This explains so much about who we are, our childhood, our family" (p. 45). Her sister Lara tells her, "It's not just about *them*! ... It's about *us*! About who *we* are!" (p. 159).[6] The prospect of explaining who she is leads Helen to embrace her Jewishness:

> I had to admit, I wanted to be Jewish — if for no other reason than because it simply made *sense*. I began to recognize myself as a person with roots and a past, with a family history, with an identity. The stories of my childhood suddenly took on new meaning — everything seemed to be shifting, an underground movement of tectonic plates slowly clicking into place, finally *fitting*. [p. 32]

When it comes to explaining how things suddenly began to fit, however, Helen can offer little more than clichés about "cultural" Jewishness. Voicing her first suspicions to her mother, she says, "I don't know why ... but I have the feeling that I'm Jewish":

> "Like that time," I said, "I went to visit Rachel after my first year of law school." Rachel's mother was a Jewish Holocaust survivor. I'd spent a weekend at their house twelve years earlier. "Remember what I told you when I came back? That it was just like being at home. With her father listening to a violin concerto in the other room, and the living room filled with books, and all her mother's plants in the window. And we sat at the kitchen counter, Rachel and her mother and I, and sipped coffee and talked and talked — and for a moment I thought I was with you and Dad — it was so much like *home*. I can't explain it — but I remember I told you about it — there was a deep resonance somehow." [pp. 24-25]

After these suspicions are confirmed,

> Lara and I laughed with recognition: the challah bread of our youth ... the smoked fish that my father loved; potato pancakes. The matzos that we had always eaten at Easter. [pp. 34-35]

These passages fall flat. It's hard to believe that Helen gained much self-understanding from recognizing that her family's potato pancakes were latkes.

---

6 Helen tells her aunt, "We needed to know about this, to understand our family, to know who we are" (p. 321).

Similarly, Helen describes her parents' past at a level of detail that cannot be relevant to her self-understanding. Why does it matter to her that her grandfather was a rabbi? I can hardly believe that his membership in the clergy left any mark on Helen herself. Indeed, very little of her parents' life as Jews left any mark, precisely because they suppressed, repressed, and forgot it. Yet Helen herself regards it as worth reporting that her mother's family in Poland lit Sabbath candles, and that her grandmother shaved her head and wore a wig.

I doubt whether Helen's detailed reconstruction of her parents' past actually accounts for anything significant about herself or her childhood. When Helen says, "I began to recognize myself as a person with roots and a past, with a family history, with an identity," I suspect that she is describing, not a recognition of who or what she already was, but a fresh *cognition* of herself, as having some roots or other, some past or other, some history or other — and hence some identity or other — where previously she had nothing at all, because of the regime of repression in which she grew up. Embracing Judaism may not be a way of recovering a pre-existing identity; it may rather be an attempt to construct an identity for the first time.

What shaped Helen as a child may have been no more than the fact that her parents had lived through persecution and loss, ultimately emerging with an iron determination to leave it all behind. Helen was also shaped, I think, by inheriting characteristics of her parents that made them survivors, starting with the sheer will to survive but also including, for example, a remarkable facility with languages, which enabled them to pass themselves off as Germans or Italians; an insight into others' motivations, which enabled them to recognize who could and could not be trusted; a capacity for self-denial and self-control; and, finally, a talent for composing stories. In writing her book, I would say, Helen was employing a gift for self-narration that she had inherited from parents who self-narrated their way out of Nazi Europe.[7] And in fashioning her new identity as a Jew, she was employing the gift that enabled her parents to fashion their identities as Catholics, with the difference that Helen was aiming for consistency with an actual past. In achieving consistency with that past, however, Helen was not necessarily achieving consistency with a pre-existent self.

---

7   Helen says that her mother escaped from the Nazis by "making up stories to save her life, spinning a tale of herself, shifting colors and sequences to suit her needs. She had invented herself a hundred times over by the time the war was over" (p. 47).

Helen embellishes the narrative of her parents' history with rich fictional details, as she herself reveals. In the midst of a fifteen-page narration of her mother's escape from Poland, she remarks:

> I don't know if he said this. I don't know Polish, or Yiddish, or whatever language they spoke to each other. I wasn't there. My mother didn't tell me. The way she told the story was like this: "And so I cut my hair short, dressed up as an Italian soldier, and marched out of Poland with the Italian army." [pp. 233-234][8]

Introducing the narration of her father's arrest, she says:

> It's not clear exactly what happened. But nothing is ever exactly clear. History is a card table full of illusions, and we must sort through and pick the ones we wish to believe. And so I choose this one. [p. 130]

When Helen says, "I choose this one," she is speaking of one among many versions of a particular episode, but the same statement applies to her entire project. Her book is subtitled "a memoir", but the story is not her own: she has appropriated it — chosen it — as the narrative on which to found a self-conception. And this appropriation raises the question of Helen's right to tell a story that had been buried by its actual protagonists.

Maybe by embellishing her parents' story, Helen gains the right to tell it, because it is now partly her creation. And maybe by revealing that the story is partly her creation, she blunts her parents' objections to its being told. For when she confesses to embellishing some parts of the story, she casts doubt over every part, any one of which could be fictional, for all the reader can tell. Once she has undermined her own credibility with the reader, she can no longer give the reader credible information about her parents. She thereby cloaks her parents in the reader's confusion about what to believe.

More pressing than the question of Helen's right to publish the story is the question of her right to confront her parents with repressed details of their past. Her mother implores her not to do the same to her Italian aunt, but she goes ahead anyway. These confrontations can seem like paternalistic "interventions" of the sort that are partly benevolent and partly hostile. It's as if Helen is punishing her elders for keeping secrets from her, by forcing them to face the secrets that they have been keeping from themselves.

---

8   Also: "I can't explain it, and I won't stop trying. I will fill this vacuum with words until I recognize them as memory" (p. 186).

That repression is enacted in the crucial scene, as Helen and her sister Lara reveal the fate of their grandparents:

"I wrote away for information," Lara said, "and I got back documentation about our family. We know what happened to your parents. We know what happened to Dad's mother."

"What happened?" my mother suddenly cried. Her hands started trembling with a terrible urgency, while her face remained frozen — a wide-eyed mask of incomprehension. "Then you know more than I do!" she exclaimed.

Lara nodded slowly, confused by my mother's sudden shift from anger to bewilderment.

"Tell me," my mother cried. "What happened? I don't even know what happened to my parents!" She turned desperately from Lara to me and back again, her hands shaking. "What happened?"

I hadn't been prepared for this. I had expected my mother to refuse to talk about it; I had been prepared for her to deny it, to get angry, to scoff at me and dismiss it, but I did not expect her to beg us to tell her how her parents were killed.

"Tell me!" my mother repeated. "What happened to them?"

I screwed up my courage, looked directly in my mother's eyes, and spoke as calmly as I could: "We found out," I said evenly, "that your parents were gassed at Belzec."

My sentence dropped like a bomb into a terrible silence. I bit my tongue. I hadn't meant to be so blunt, so harsh. Lara kicked me under the table, and with growing panic I waited for my mother's reaction. Seconds ticked by, and I was consumed by an excruciating sense of guilt that I had just shattered my mother's world.

But my mother did not react. She stared at me with the same puzzled look on her face, as if I hadn't spoken. "Tell me what happened to them," she repeated, hands outstretched.

I kept quiet, shaken. I can't continue with this, I thought. I can't bear to do this …

"I don't even know what happened to my parents!" Mom cried. "Tell me!" [pp. 42-43]

"My sentence dropped like a bomb into a terrible silence," Helen says. Her mother had always dismissed questions about the fate of her parents by saying, cryptically, that they had died "in a bomb". Helen is now, so to speak, killing her grandparents all over again, by dropping a verbal bomb. She drops it into "a terrible silence", a brief fragment of the "long silence" that had enabled her mother to un-know her parents' deaths. And Helen's mother bravely persists — perseverates — in not knowing.

At the end of the book, Helen is visiting her Aunt Zosia in Rome, writing the book. So she is simultaneously writing the story and living what she writes. On the same visit, she reveals her discoveries about the family to her Roman cousin and faces the ire of her aunt for doing so.

The reader wonders to what extent the writing of this chapter influenced the living of it — to what extent it was lived so as to be written. Did Helen tell her cousin of his Jewish background for independent reasons, or she did tell him in order to write about it? And this question, raised by her contemporaneous narration of writing the book, echoes back through the preceding chapters. How much of her research was undertaken by the daughter and how much by the aspiring writer? In plotting with her sister to pry information out of their parents, was she also plotting her memoir?

Could it be that Helen came out as a lesbian in order to have the parallel story lines of uncovering her parents' secret and disclosing her own? Her mother refuses to believe that Helen is a lesbian, just as she refuses to take in the revelation of her parents' murder. As they say, you couldn't make that up — unless, of course, you made it up in order to make it happen in order to write it.

Or maybe it's the reverse. Maybe Helen wrote it in order to motivate herself to make it happen. In writing the book, she wrote herself into a corner, so to speak, since her friends and lovers would see the hypocrisy of her remaining closeted while outing her parents. How better to resolve her own indecision about whether to come out?

Or maybe Helen just researched her parents' past, came out as a lesbian, and wrote a book about it all.

After Long Silence is a book of stories about silence. Silence is the villain of the piece. The human villains, Nazis and Bolsheviks, make only the briefest appearance. Even Helen's description of the Petlura Days pogrom in Lvov, as witnessed by her mother and aunt, reaches its climax in Helen's own unwillingness to ask her mother whether she was raped. In a scene of horrors, silence takes center stage.

The book has many heroes: Helen's father and mother, and those who helped them to escape. But the real hero of the book is the narrated truth, which triumphs over silence in the end. The book is one long testament to the healing power of The True Story.

Yet with some truths, there is nothing to do but forget. I believe in virtuous Holocaust deniers — namely, the survivors, many of whom, like

Helen's parents, managed to achieve a merciful forgetfulness. "Forget the past, live for the future," Helen's mother says. Hers was a past worth forgetting.

Once remembered, some of her mother's past can be domesticated by being told as a story, especially since it has an outwardly happy ending. But one part cannot be told as a story, because it has no narrative ending. It goes: "And so they were herded into a windowless chamber and gassed to death." One cannot imagine punctuating that sentence with "The End". It's a finish that isn't an ending, because it brings no closure. In the minds of the survivors, the final scene never ends.

Surely, this narratively intractable passage of history is the one that Helen's mother is struggling hardest to repress. Helen can't domesticate it for her, and so I continue to wonder whether she was entitled to tell it at all.

As for Helen's right to publish the story, she says that she is honoring her forgotten ancestors and expressing love for her parents:

> My family is greater than just my parents and Zosia — my family extends backward in time and space. I want to put them on record, however imperfectly — I want them to be seen and heard.
>
> And strangely enough, on the page I begin to recognize myself in my parents — a gesture here, a question there. My attachment to them grows stronger with each sentence that arranges itself before me. Perhaps this is the ultimate irony of my family: I express my love for them in ways that are invariably the opposite of what they would wish. [p. 318]

A complicated passage. The declaration of wanting her relatives to be seen and heard is an implicit rebuke to her parents, survivors who did not bear witness for the dead: they lived to tell the tale and then refused to tell it. Helen then disclaims responsibility for this rebuke: the sentences arrange themselves on the page, she says, as if the tale is telling itself. Finally, she expresses the mixed motives behind the whole complicated project, an expression of love that is also an expression of defiance.

I believe Helen when she says that writing her book is an expression of love; I believe the same of her family interventions. Still, I finished the book wishing to know more about how her parents received it. We are told only that they did not approve. As for the details, Helen is silent.

When I was a child, I was told that my father's sister Emma had perished in the Holocaust. That phrase made the Holocaust sound like a vortex into which people just disappeared, like sailors who are said to have perished at sea. The poetic vagueness of it expressed my father's perfect ignorance as to when, where, and how his sister had died.

When Germany invaded Western Europe in May of 1940, Emma was living with her husband and young daughter in the Dutch village of Borculo, which was close to the German border and immediately overrun. My father was living in Antwerp and was able to escape, together with his other sister, Molly, and their parents. They made their way through France and Spain to Portugal, and thence to the United States, where my father spent the war working for the O.S.S. in Washington, D.C. He traveled to Borculo immediately after the war, on one of the first postwar visas issued to civilians. When he knocked on the door of Emma's house, he found strangers sitting at her table, eating from her dishes — and claiming never to have heard of her.

In the early 1990s, an amateur genealogist in Holland wrote to my father in New York and to me in Ann Arbor, Michigan, seeking information about people with the last name of Velleman. He told us what he already knew about my father's family history, including many names and dates that my father could confirm. He also included information that my father had not previously known — in particular, the names of the camps where various aunts, uncles, and cousins had been killed, and the dates of their deaths. No such information was included for Emma, but we reasoned that information about Emma's death might have eluded his researches because it was recorded under her married name. My father wrote back, supplying Emma's particulars and asking the genealogist to apply his methods to the question of her fate.

One day my father called to say that a letter had arrived from our correspondent in Holland. He then began to read: Emma, her husband, and their daughter had been interned at the concentration camp Westerbork, in Holland; they had been placed on a transport bound for Auschwitz on November 24, 1942; and the mother and daughter were presumed to have died on arrival, three days later. My father began to sob and dropped the phone. I had never before heard my father cry.

When my parents next visited Ann Arbor, my father silently handed me a manila folder full of yellowed correspondence. It had been given to him by his surviving sister, Molly, when he told her what he had learned about Emma and her family. In the years immediately following the war, Molly had corresponded with international relief agencies on behalf of the family in America, seeking information, in particular, about Emma's daughter, Rita, who might have survived without knowing how to contact her relatives. The folder now handed to me by my father contained carbon copies of Molly's inquiries, along with the original replies. The latter were all dead-ends, with one exception. A letter from the International Red Cross, dated 1955, informed the family that Rita had been interned in the concentration camp Westerbork, in Holland; had been placed on a transport bound for Auschwitz on November 24, 1942; and was presumed to have died on arrival, three days later.

So my father had known Emma's fate all along. Why, I asked, had he recruited the genealogist to investigate what he already knew? Why had he reacted to the information as if hearing it for the first time?

He replied, "I had repressed it."

When I was a teenager, I quizzed my father about the war, and he told me the story of his escape: the chance encounter with a rich uncle who owned a car, which carried the family to safety; the time in Bordeaux when he helped stamp passports for the Portuguese consul who was defying orders from Lisbon by issuing transit visas to thousands of refugees; the night they spent in a broken-down castle where the beds were full of lice; how he and his mother crossed the Spanish border on foot, mopping their brows with handkerchiefs holding diamonds from his father's workshop. (My grandfather was a diamond cleaver, and his occupation was noted in his passport, so that he would be searched.) My father also told me about his trip back to Europe after the war — a long story, mainly about coincidental meetings on board ship.

After learning how he had repressed his knowledge of Emma's death, I realized that my father had turned his wartime experiences into a picaresque. Yes, his sister and her family had perished — he told that, too, though not, of course, the details that he had not yet recovered. But the central, significant event was lost in a series of adventures, all of which were bathed in the glow of a happy ending on the horizon.

Our brush with genealogy prompted me to start researching the family's history. This was just a few years before the Internet transformed genealogical research, and so I spent many hours in the basement of the local Mormon center, reeling through microfilmed records of mysterious Mormon rites performed for my ancestors. Like Helen Fremont, I had found religion, though in my case, it wasn't Judaism.

Also like Helen Fremont, I was taking on the self-image of the so-called second generation, whose childhoods were touched in some way by their parents' brush with the Holocaust. And I was adopting that self-image by hitching my life story to that of my father and, more importantly, to that of his sister Emma, whom I could never know. I even visited Borculo during a break from a conference in the Netherlands. But what is it to me, what is it about me, that I had an aunt who died in Auschwitz ten years before I was born?

I think that the death of my aunt is meaningful to me because she meant so much to my father, who meant so much to me. I would like to say that I grieve for her in solidarity with him, but the fact is that I doubt whether he ever really grieved for her. I once asked my father whether, after receiving confirmation of her death, the family had held a memorial of any kind. The idea had never occurred to him.

So I suspect that my father passed on to me an emotional task that he could not bear to do himself. And I suspect that Helen Fremont was given a much heavier emotional task, with the added burden of not knowing what it was. In this sense, discovering her parents' history really was a discovery of her own identity, after all. She was Jewish despite her Catholic upbringing because she was carrying the unresolved grief of Jewish parents for grandparents who were murdered for being Jews. Even if our parents don't pass on their stories, they still pass on emotions that only their stories can help us to resolve. To that extent, at least, their stories are ours.

Bibliography

Ackerman, Felicia. "No, Thanks, I Don't Want to Die with Dignity". *Providence Journal-Bulletin*, April 19, 1990.

—. "Assisted Suicide, Terminal Illness, Severe Disability, and the Double Standard". In *Physician-Assisted Suicide: Expanding the Debate*, ed. Margaret P. Battin, Rosamond Rhodes, and Anita Silvers. New York: Routledge, 1998, pp. 149-161.

Adams, Robert Merrihew. "Existence, Self-Interest, and the Problem of Evil". *Noûs* 13 (1979): 53-65. http://dx.doi.org/10.2307/2214795

Allen, Woody, director. *Everything You Always Wanted to Know About Sex* But Were Afraid to Ask*. Rollins-Joffe Productions, United Artists, 1972.

Anderson, Elizabeth. *Value in Ethics and Economics*. Cambridge, MA: Harvard University Press, 1993.

Benatar, David. "Why It Is Better Never to Come Into Existence". *American Philosophical Quarterly* 34 (1997): 345-355.

Berenson, Bernard. *Sketch for a Self Portrait*. London: Robin Clark, 1991.

Bigelow, John, John Campbell, and Robert Pargetter. "Death and Well-Being". *Pacific Philosophical Quarterly* 71 (1990): 119.

Blyth, Eric, Marilyn Crawshaw, Jean Haase, and Jennifer Speirs. "The Implications of Adoption for Donor Offspring Following Donor-Assisted Conception". *Child & Family Social Work* 6 (2001): 295-304. http://dx.doi.org/10.1046/j.1365-2206.2001.00214.x

Blyth, Eric, Marilyn Crawshaw, and Jennifer Speirs, editors. *Truth and the Child 10 Years On: Information Exchange in Donor Assisted Conception*. Birmingham: British Association of Social Workers, 1998.

Blyth, Eric, and Abigail Farrand. "Anonymity in Donor-Assisted Conception and the UN Convention on the Rights of the Child". *The International Journal of Children's Rights* 12 (2004): 89-104. http://dx.doi.org/10.1163/1571818041904290

Bouchard, Thomas J., Jr. "Genetic Influence on Human Psychological Traits: A Survey". *Current Directions in Psychological Science* 13 (2004): 148-151. http://dx.doi.org/10.1111/j.0963-7214.2004.00295.x

Brandt, Richard B. "Two Concepts of Utility". In *The Limits of Utilitarianism*, ed. Harlan B. Miller and William H. Williams. Minneapolis: University of Minnesota Press, 1982, pp. 169-185.

Brock, Dan W. "Voluntary Active Euthanasia". *The Hastings Center Report* 22 (1992): 10-22. http://dx.doi.org/10.2307/3562560. Reprinted in *Life and Death: Philosophical Essays in Biomedical Ethics*. Cambridge: Cambridge University Press, 1993, pp. 202-234.

Brodt, Susan E., and Philip G. Zimbardo. "Modifying Shyness-Related Social Behavior Through Symptom Misattribution". *Journal of Personality and Social Psychology* 41 (1981): 437-449. http://dx.doi.org/10.1037/0022-3514.41.3.437

Brodzinsky, David M. "A Stress and Coping Model of Adoption Adjustment". In *The Psychology of Adoption*, ed. David M. Brodzinsky and Marshall D. Schechter. New York: Oxford University Press, 1990, pp. 3-24.

Bruce, Nigel, Ann K. Mitchell, and Kate Priestley. *Truth and the Child: A Contribution to the Debate on the Warnock Report*. Edinburgh: Family Care, 1988.

Camus, Albert. "The Myth of Sisyphus". In *The Myth of Sisyphus and Other Essays*, translated by Justin O'Brien. New York: Vintage Books, 1956, pp. 88-91.

Cassell, Eric J. "Recognizing Suffering". *The Hastings Center Report* 21 (1991): 24-31. http://dx.doi.org/10.2307/3563319

Charmaz, Kathy. "Loss of Self: A Fundamental Form of Suffering in the Chronically Ill". *Sociology of Health & Illness* 5 (1983): 168-195. http://dx.doi.org/10.1111/1467-9566.ep10491512

Csikszentmihalyi, Mihaly. *Flow: The Psychology of Optimal Experience*. New York: Harper & Row, 1990.

D'Arms, Justin, and Daniel Jacobson. "The Moralistic Fallacy: On the 'Appropriateness' of Emotions". *Philosophy and Phenomenological Research* 61 (2000): 65-90. http://dx.doi.org/10.2307/2653403

Darwall, Stephen L. "Self-Interest and Self-Concern". *Social Philosophy and Policy* 14 (1997): 158-178. http://dx.doi.org/10.1017/s0265052500001710. Reprinted in *Self-Interest*, ed. Ellen Paul. Cambridge: Cambridge University Press, 1997.

—. *Welfare and Rational Care*. Princeton, NJ: Princeton University Press, 2004.

Dennett, Daniel C. "The Origins of Selves". *Cogito* 3 (1989): 163-173. http://dx.doi.org/10.5840/cogito19893348

—. "The Reality of Selves". In *Consciousness Explained*. Boston: Little, Brown and Company, 1991, pp. 412-430.

—. "The Self as the Center of Narrative Gravity". In *Self and Consciousness: Multiple Perspectives*, ed. Frank S. Kessel, Pamela M. Cole, and Dale L. Johnson. Hillsdale, NJ: Erlbaum Associates, 1992, pp. 103-115.

Duclos, Sandra E., James D. Laird, Eric Schneider, Melissa Sexter, Lisa Stern, and Oliver Van Lighten. "Emotion-Specific Effects of Facial Expressions and Postures on Emotional Experience". *Journal of Personality and Social Psychology* 57 (1989): 100-108. http://dx.doi.org/10.1037//0022-3514.57.1.100

Dutton, Donald G., and Arthur P. Aron. "Some Evidence for Heightened Sexual Attraction Under Conditions of High Anxiety". *Journal of Personality and Social Psychology* 30 (1974): 510-517. http://dx.doi.org/10.1037/h0037031

Dworkin, Gerald. "Is More Choice Better Than Less?". *Midwest Studies in Philosophy* 7 (1982): 47-61. http://dx.doi.org/10.1111/j.1475-4975.1982.tb00083.x

Dworkin, Ronald, Thomas Nagel, Robert Nozick, John Rawls, Thomas Scanlon, and Judith Jarvis Thomson. "Assisted Suicide: The Philosophers' Brief". *The New York Review of Books* 44 (1997): 41-47.

Eccleston, Christopher. "The Attentional Control of Pain: Methodological and Theoretical Concerns". *Pain* 63 (1995): 3-10. http://dx.doi.org/10.1016/0304-3959(95)00093-8

Feinberg, Joel. *Harm to Others*. New York: Oxford University Press, 1984.

Feldman, Fred. "Some Puzzles About the Evil of Death". *The Philosophical Review* 100 (1991): 225-227. http://dx.doi.org/10.2307/2185300

Frankfurt, Harry G. "The Problem of Action". *American Philosophical Quarterly* 15 (1978): 157-162. Reprinted in *The Importance of What We Care About*. Cambridge: Cambridge University Press, 1988, pp. 69-79. http://dx.doi.org/10.1017/cbo9780511818172

—. "The Importance of What We Care About". In *The Importance of What We Care About*. Cambridge: Cambridge University Press, 1988, pp. 80-94.

—. "On the Usefulness of Final Ends". In *Necessity, Volition, and Love*. Cambridge: Cambridge University Press, 1999, pp. 82-94. http://dx.doi.org/10.1017/cbo9780511624643

—. "On Caring". In *Necessity, Volition, and Love*, pp. 155-180.

—. "The Dear Self". *Philosophers' Imprint* 1 (2001): 1-14, http://www.philosophersimprint.org/001000/

Freeman, Michael. "The New Birth Right? Identity and the Child of the Reproduction Revolution". *The International Journal of Children's Rights* 4 (1996): 273-297. http://dx.doi.org/10.1163/157181896x00176

Fremont, Helen. *After Long Silence: A Memoir*. New York: Dell Publishing, 1999.

Frith, Lucy. "Gamete Donation and Anonymity: The Ethical and Legal Debate". *Human Reproduction* 16 (2001): 818-824. http://dx.doi.org/10.1093/humrep/16.5.818

Gendler, Tamar Szabó. "Personal Identity and Thought-Experiments". *The Philosophical Quarterly* 52 (2002): 34-54. http://dx.doi.org/10.1111/1467-9213.00251

Gibbard, Allan. *Thinking How to Live*. Cambridge, MA: Harvard University Press, 2003.

Gollancz, David. "Give Me My Own History". *The Guardian*, May 19, 2002.

Govier, Trudy. "What Should We Do About Future People?". *American Philosophical Quarterly* 16 (1979): 105-113.

Griffin, James. *Well-Being: Its Meaning, Measurement, and Moral Importance*. Oxford: Clarendon Press, 1986.

Hamlyn, D. W. "The Phenomena of Love and Hate". *Philosophy* 53 (1978): 5-20. http://dx.doi.org/10.1017/s0031819100016272

Hanser, Matthew. "Harming Future People". *Philosophy & Public Affairs* 19 (1990): 47-70.

Hare, Caspar. "Voices from Another World: Must We Respect the Interests of People Who Do Not, and Will Never, Exist?". *Ethics* 117 (2007): 498-523. http://dx.doi.org/10.1086/512172

Haslanger, Sally. "Persistence Through Time". In *The Oxford Handbook of Metaphysics*, ed. Michael J. Loux and Dean W. Zimmerman. Oxford: Oxford University Press, 2005, pp. 315-354. http://dx.doi.org/10.1093/oxfordhb/9780199284221.001.0001

Herman, Barbara. *Moral Literacy*. Cambridge, MA: Harvard University Press, 2007, pp. 13-18.

Hill, Thomas E., Jr. "Self-Regarding Suicide: A Modified Kantian View". In *Autonomy and Self-Respect*. Cambridge: Cambridge University Press, 1991, pp. 85-103.

Hodgkin, Rachel, and Peter Newell. *Implementation Handbook for the Convention on the Rights of the Child*. New York: UNICEF, revised edn 2002.

Hofweber, Thomas, and J. David Velleman. "How to Endure". *Philosophical Quarterly* 61 (2011): 37-57. http://dx.doi.org/10.1111/j.1467-9213.2010.671.x

Jeshion, Robin. "Acquaintanceless *De Re* Belief". In *Meaning and Truth: Investigations in Philosophical Semantics*, ed. Joseph Keim Campbell, Michael O'Rourke, and David Shier. New York: Seven Bridges Press, 2002, pp. 53-74.

Johnston, Mark. "The Authority of Affect". *Philosophy and Phenomenological Research* 63 (2001): 181-214. http://dx.doi.org/10.1111/j.1933-1592.2001.tb00097.x

Kamisar, Yale. "Euthanasia Legislation: Some Non-Religious Objections". In *Euthanasia and the Right to Die*, ed. A. B. Downing. New York: Humanities Press, 1970, pp. 85-133.

Kamm, Frances. "A Right to Choose Death?". *Boston Review* 22 (1997): 20-23.

—. "Physician-Assisted Suicide, the Doctrine of Double Effect, and the Ground of Value". *Ethics* 109 (1999): 586-605. http://dx.doi.org/10.1086/233923

Kant, Immanuel. *Groundwork of the Metaphysic of Morals*, translated by H. J. Paton. New York: Harper & Row, 1964.

Kavka, Gregory S. "The Paradox of Future Individuals". *Philosophy & Public Affairs* 11 (1982): 93-112.

Keller, Simon. "Presentism and Truthmaking". In *Oxford Studies in Metaphysics*, vol. I, ed. Dean W. Zimmerman. Oxford: Oxford University Press, 2004, pp. 83-106. http://dx.doi.org/10.1093/acprof:oso/9780199603039.001.0001

Koenig, Laura B., and Thomas J. Bouchard, Jr. "Genetic and Environmental Influences on the Traditional Moral Values Triad — Authoritarianism,

Conservatism, and Religiousness — as Assessed by Quantitative Behavior Genetic Methods". In *Where God and Science Meet: How Brain and Evolutionary Studies Alter Our Understanding of Religion, Volume I: Evolution, Genes, and the Religious Brain*, ed. Patrick McNamara. Westport, CT: Praeger, 2006, pp. 31-60.

Kolodny, Niko. "Love as Valuing a Relationship". *The Philosophical Review* 112 (2003): 135-189. http://dx.doi.org/10.1215/00318108-112-2-135

Korsgaard, Christine M. *The Sources of Normativity*, ed. Onora. Cambridge: Cambridge University Press, 1996.

—. "Self-Constitution: Action, Identity, and Integrity". The Locke Lectures, 2002.

Kumar, Rahul. "Who Can Be Wronged?". *Philosophy & Public Affairs* 31 (2003): 99-118. http://dx.doi.org/10.1111/j.1088-4963.2003.00099.x

Laing, Jacqueline A., and David S. Oderberg. "Artificial Reproduction, the 'Welfare Principle', and the Common Good". *Medical Law Review* 13 (2005): 328-356. http://dx.doi.org/10.1093/medlaw/fwi022

Laird, James D. "The Real Role of Facial Response in the Experience of Emotion: A Reply to Tourangeau and Ellsworth, and Others". *Journal of Personality and Social Psychology* 47 (1984): 909-917. http://dx.doi.org/10.1037//0022-3514.47.4.909

Lewis, Clarence Irving. *An Analysis of Knowledge and Valuation*. La Salle, IL: Open Court Publishing Company, 1946.

Lewis, David K. "Survival and Identity". In *The Identities of Persons*, ed. Amélie Oksenberg Rorty, Berkeley, CA: University of California Press, 1976, pp. 17-40. Reprinted in *Philosophical Papers*, vol. I, Oxford: Oxford University Press, 1983, pp. 55-77.

MacIntyre, Alasdair. *After Virtue: A Study in Moral Theory*. Notre Dame, IN: University of Notre Dame Press, 1984.

McCracken, Lance M., James W. Carson, Christopher Eccleston, and Francis J. Keefe. "Acceptance and Change in the Context of Chronic Pain". *Pain* 109 (2004): 4-7.

McCracken, Lance M., and Chris Eccleston. "Coping or Acceptance: What to Do About Chronic Pain?". *Pain* 105 (2003): 197-204. http://dx.doi.org/10.1016/s0304-3959(03)00202-1

McMahan, Jefferson. "Preventing the Existence of People with Disabilities". In *Quality of Life and Human Difference: Genetic Testing, Health Care, and Disability*, ed. David Wasserman, Jerome Bickenbach, and Robert Wachbroit. New York: Cambridge University Press, 2005, pp. 142-171.

McTaggart, J. Ellis. "The Unreality of Time". *Mind* 17 (1908): 457-474. http://dx.doi.org/10.1093/mind/xvii.4.457

McWhinnie, Alexina. "Gamete Donation and Anonymity: Should Offspring from Donated Gametes Continue to Be Denied Knowledge of Their Origins and Antecedents?". *Human Reproduction* 16 (2001): 807-817. http://dx.doi.org/10.1093/humrep/16.5.807

Merleau-Ponty, Maurice. *Phenomenology of Perception*, translated by Colin Smith. London: Routledge and Kegan Paul, 1962, pp. 411-412. Reprinted in *Maurice Merleau-Ponty: Basic Writings*, ed. Thomas Baldwin. London: Routledge, 2003, pp. 62-233. http://dx.doi.org/10.4324/9780203502532

Moore, G. E. *Plural and Conflicting Values*. Oxford: Oxford University Press, 1990.

Müller, Ulrich, and Barbara Perry. "Adopted Persons' Search for and Contact with Their Birth Parents I: Who Searches and Why?". *Adoption Quarterly* 4 (2001): 5-37. http://dx.doi.org/10.1300/j145v04n03_02

Murdoch, Iris. "The Sublime and the Good". In *Existentialists and Mystics: Writings on Philosophy and Literature*, ed. Peter Conradi. New York: Penguin, 1997, pp. 205-220.

Nagel, Thomas. "Death". In *Mortal Questions*. New York: Cambridge University Press, 1991.

—. "The Fragmentation of Value". In *Mortal Questions*.

Nehamas, Alexander. *Nietzsche: Life as Literature*. Cambridge, MA: Harvard University Press, 1985.

Nickman, Steven L. "Retroactive Loss in Adopted Persons". In *Continuing Bonds: New Understandings of Grief*, ed. Dennis Klass, Phyllis R. Silverman, and Steven Nickman. Washington, DC: Taylor & Francis, 1996, pp. 257-272. http://dx.doi.org/10.4324/9781315800790

Parfit, Derek. "Personal Identity". *The Philosophical Review* 80 (1971): 3-27. http://dx.doi.org/10.2307/2184309

—. "On Doing the Best for Our Children". In *Ethics and Population*, ed. Michael D. Bayles. Cambridge, MA: Schenkman, 1976, pp. 100-115.

—. *Reasons and Persons*. Oxford: Oxford University Press, 1984.

Perry, John. "Belief and Acceptance". In *The Problem of the Essential Indexical and Other Essays*. New York: Oxford University Press, 1993, pp. 53-68.

Plotz, David. *The Genius Factory: The Curious History of the Nobel Prize Sperm Bank*. New York: Random House, 2005.

Railton, Peter. "Facts and Values". *Philosophical Topics* 14 (1986): 5-31. http://dx.doi.org/10.5840/philtopics19861421

—. "Moral Realism". *The Philosophical Review* 95 (1986): 163-207. http://dx.doi.org/10.2307/2185589

Rosati, Connie S. "Darwall on Welfare and Rational Care". *Philosophical Studies* 30 (2006): 619-635.

—. "Mortality, Agency, and Regret". *Poznań Studies in the Philosophy of the Sciences and the Humanities* 94 (2007): 231-259.

Russell, Bertrand. *The Philosophy of Logical Atomism*. Abingdon: Routledge Classics, 2010.

Schelling, Thomas C. *The Strategy of Conflict*. Cambridge, MA: Harvard University Press, 1960.

—. "Strategic Relationships in Dying". In *Choice and Consequence: Perspectives of an Errant Economist*. Cambridge, MA: Harvard University Press, 1984, pp. 147-157.

Schwartz, Thomas. "Obligations to Posterity". In *Obligations to Future Generations*, ed. R. I. Sikora and Brian Barry. Philadelphia: Temple University Press, 1978, pp. 3-13.

Sen, Amartya. "Utilitarianism and Welfarism". *The Journal of Philosophy* 76 (1979): 463-489. http://dx.doi.org/10.2307/2025934

—. "Plural Utility". *Proceedings of the Aristotelian Society* 81 (1980-1981): 202-204.

—. "Moral Information", the first lecture in "Well-Being, Agency and Freedom: The Dewey Lectures 1984". *The Journal of Philosophy* 82 (1985): 169-221. http://dx.doi.org/10.2307/2026184

—. "Well-Being and Freedom", the second lecture in "Well-Being, Agency and Freedom". *The Journal of Philosophy* 82 (1985): 169-221.

Shiffrin, Seana Valentine. "Wrongful Life, Procreative Responsibility, and the Significance of Harm". *Legal Theory* 5 (1999): 117-148. http://dx.doi.org/10.1017/s1352325299052015

Sidgwick, Henry. *The Methods of Ethics*. Indianapolis: Hackett Publishing, 1981.

Slote, Michael. "Goods and Lives". *Pacific Philosophical Quarterly* 63 (1982): 311-326.

Stell, Lance K. "Dueling and the Right to Life". *Ethics* 90 (1979): 7-26. http://dx.doi.org/10.1086/292130

Taylor, Charles. *Sources of the Self: The Making of the Modern Identity*. Cambridge, MA: Harvard University Press, 1989.

Temkin, Larry S. "Intransitivity and the Mere Addition Paradox". *Philosophy & Public Affairs* 16 (1987): 138-187.

Tooley, Michael. "Value, Obligation and the Asymmetry Question". *Bioethics* 12 (1998): 111-124. http://dx.doi.org/10.1111/1467-8519.00099

Torek, Paul Volkening. *Something to Look Forward To: Personal Identity, Prudence, and Ethics*. Ph.D. dissertation, University of Michigan, 1995.

Turner, A. J. and A. Coyle. "What Does It Mean to Be a Donor Offspring? The Identity Experiences of Adults Conceived by Donor Insemination and the Implications for Counselling and Therapy". *Human Reproduction* 15 (2000): 2041-2051. http://dx.doi.org/10.1093/humrep/15.9.2041

Velleman, J. David. "Well-Being and Time". *Pacific Philosophical Quarterly* 72 (1991): 48-77.

—. "Against the Right to Die". *The Journal of Medicine & Philosophy* 17 (1992): 665-681. http://dx.doi.org/10.1093/jmp/17.6.665. Revised version in the 2nd edn of *Ethics in Practice: An Anthology*, ed. Hugh LaFollette. Chichester: John Wiley & Sons, 2014, pp. 96-100.

—. "What Happens When Someone Acts?". *Mind* 101 (1992): 461-481. http://dx.doi. org/10.1093/mind/101.403.461. Reprinted in *The Possibility of Practical Reason*, 2nd edn. Ann Arbor, MI: Maize Books, 2015, pp. 100-123.

—. "Self to Self". *Philosophical Review* 105 (1996): 39-76. Reprinted in *Self to Self: Selected Essays*. Cambridge: Cambridge University Press, 2005, pp. 170-202. http://dx.doi.org/10.1017/cbo9780511498862

—. "A Right of Self-Termination?". *Ethics* 109 (1999): 606-628. http://dx.doi. org/10.1086/233924

—. "Love as a Moral Emotion". *Ethics* 109 (1999): 338-374. http://dx.doi. org/10.1086/233898. Reprinted in *Self to Self*, pp. 70-109.

—. "The Voice of Conscience". *Proceedings of the Aristotelian Society* 99 (1999): 57-76. Reprinted in *Self to Self*, pp. 110-128. http://dx.doi.org/10.1111/1467-9264.00045

—. "From Self Psychology to Moral Philosophy". *Nous* 34 (2000): 349-377. Reprinted in *Self to Self*, pp. 224-252.

—. "Identification and Identity". In *The Contours of Agency: Essays on Themes from Harry Frankfurt*, ed. Sarah Buss and Lee Overton. Cambridge, MA: MIT Press, 2002, pp. 91-128. Reprinted in *Self to Self*, pp. 330-360.

—. "Motivation by Ideal". *Philosophical Explorations* 5 (2002): 89-103. http://dx.doi. org/10.1080/10002002058538724. Reprinted in *Self to Self*, pp. 312-329.

—. "Narrative Explanation". *The Philosophical Review* 112 (2003): 1-25. http://dx.doi. org/10.1215/00318108-112-1-1

—. "Family History". *Philosophical Papers* 34 (2005): 357-378. http://dx.doi.org/ 10.1080/05568640509485163

—. "A Brief Introduction to Kantian Ethics". In *Self to Self*, pp. 16-44.

—. "So It Goes". Published online as the 2006 Amherst Lecture in Philosophy, http:// www.amherstlecture.org/velleman2006/index.html

—. "What Good is a Will?". In *Action in Context*, ed. Anton Leist. Berlin: Walter de Gruyter, 2007. Reprinted in *The Possibility of Practical Reason*, 2nd edn.

—. "Beyond Price". *Ethics* 118 (2008): pp. 306-329. http://dx.doi.org/10.1086/523746

—. "Persons in Prospect". *Philosophy & Public Affairs* 36 (2008): 221-288. http:// dx.doi.org/10.1111/j.1088-4963.2008.00139_1.x, http://dx.doi.org/10.1111/j.1088-4963.2008.00139_2.x, http://dx.doi.org/10.1111/j.1088-4963.2008.00139_3.x

—. "A Theory of Value". *Ethics* 118 (2008): 410-436. http://dx.doi.org/10.1086/528782. Reprinted in *How We Get Along*. New York: Cambridge University Press, 2009, chapter 2.

—. "The Way of the Wanton". In *Practical Identity and Narrative Agency*, ed. Kim Atkins and Catriona MacKenzie. London: Routledge, 2008, pp. 169-192. http:// dx.doi.org/10.4324/9780203937839. Reprinted in *The Possibility of Practical Reason*, 2nd edn, pp. 280-305.

—. "Reading Kant's Groundwork". In *Ethics: Essential Readings in Moral Theory*, ed. George Sher. New York: Routledge, 2012, pp. 343-359. http://dx.doi.org/10.4324/9780203723746

—. "Dying". *Think* 11 (2012): 29-32. http://dx.doi.org/10.1017/S147717561200022X

—. "The Rights to a Life". Forthcoming in *On Life-Writing*, ed. Zachary Leader. Oxford: Oxford University Press, 2015.

Vonnegut, Kurt, Jr. *Slaughterhouse-Five or, The Children's Crusade: A Duty-Dance with Death*. New York: Dell Publishing, 1969.

Weinberg, Rivka. "The Moral Complexity of Sperm Donation". *Bioethics* 22 (2008): 166-178. http://dx.doi.org/10.1111/j.1467-8519.2007.00624.x

White, Hayden. *Metahistory: The Historical Imagination in Nineteenth-Century Europe*. Baltimore: Johns Hopkins University Press, 1973.

—. *The Content of Form: Narrative Discourse and Historical Representation*. Baltimore: Johns Hopkins University Press, 1987.

—. *Tropics of Discourse: Essays in Cultural Criticism*. Baltimore: Johns Hopkins University Press, 1987.

Williams, Bernard. "Imagination and the Self". In *Problems of the Self: Philosophical Papers 1956-1972*. Cambridge: Cambridge University Press, 1973, pp. 26-45.

—. "The Makropulos Case: Reflections on the Tedium of Immortality". In *Problems of the Self*, pp. 82-100.

—. "Persons, Character and Morality". In *The Identities of Persons*, ed. Amélie Oksenberg Rorty. Berkeley, CA: University of California Press, 1976, pp. 197-216.

Index

This book need not end here...

At Open Book Publishers, we are changing the nature of the traditional academic book. The title you have just read will not be left on a library shelf, but will be accessed online by hundreds of readers each month across the globe. We make all our books free to read online so that students, researchers and members of the public who can't afford a printed edition can still have access to the same ideas as you.

Our digital publishing model also allows us to produce online supplementary material, including extra chapters, reviews, links and other digital resources. Find *Beyond Price: Essays on Life and Death* on our website to access its online extras. Please check this page regularly for ongoing updates, and join the conversation by leaving your own comments:

http://www.openbookpublishers.com/isbn/9781783741670

If you enjoyed this book, and feel that research like this should be available to all readers, regardless of their income, please think about donating to us. Our company is run entirely by academics, and our publishing decisions are based on intellectual merit and public value rather than on commercial viability. We do not operate for profit and all donations, as with all other revenue we generate, will be used to finance new Open Access publications.

For further information about what we do, how to donate to OBP, additional digital material related to our titles or to order our books, please visit our website: http://www.openbookpublishers.com

OpenBook
Publishers
Knowledge is for sharing